# REHABILITATION OF THE LOWER LIMB AMPUTEE FOR NURSES AND THERAPISTS

# Rehabilitation of the Lower Limb Amputee

For Nurses and Therapists

W. HUMM MSRG, SRRG, MISPO

*Senior Remedial Gymnast. Specialist in Amputee and Prosthetic Training, Clayton Hospital, Wakefield, West Yorkshire*

*Foreword by*

A. E. S. RAINEY MB, FRCSEd, FRCSI
*Consultant Orthopaedic Surgeon, Pinderfields Hospital, Wakefield, West Yorkshire*

THIRD EDITION

BAILLIÈRE TINDALL · LONDON

A BAILLIÈRE TINDALL book published by
Cassell & Collier Macmillan Publishers Ltd
35 Red Lion Square, London WC1R 4SG
and at Sydney, Auckland, Toronto, Johannesburg
an affiliate of
Macmillan Publishing Co. Inc.
New York


© 1977 Baillière Tindall
a division of Cassell & Collier Macmillan Publishers Ltd

First published 1965
Second edition 1969
Third edition 1977


ISBN 0 7020 0650 5

Printed in Great Britain by Butler & Tanner Ltd
Frome and London

# Contents

# Foreword

Amputation is an ancient surgical procedure with evidence of the existence of amputees among prehistoric man. Early surgical amputation was a crude affair in which the patient was not anaesthetized; the limb was rapidly removed and dipped into boiling oil, leaving a stump unsuitable even for primitive prosthesis. With the development of anaesthesia and aseptic techniques stumps could be fashioned and interest in better prostheses for amputees has increased since World War II.

The destructive nature of amputation can give rise to a defeatist attitude in which the operation is considered undesirable although necessary but the amputation of an irreparable or diseased limb should be considered rather as the first step towards returning the patient to a normal useful place in society.

Success in any surgical procedure is often a team effort and nowhere is this better illustrated than with amputations. In the early postoperative phase the cooperation between surgeon, nurse and therapist is crucial and, at a later stage, between therapist and prosthetist. It is correctly pointed out in this edition that the most important member of the team is the patient.

Early rehabilitation is essential and, where elective amputation can be performed, introduction of the patient to the Amputee Unit to see the amputees and the available prostheses before surgery is of mutual benefit both to the patient and the therapist.

The first part of this revised edition has been largely rewritten, setting out clearly the modern concepts of levels of amputation linked to prosthetic requirements. The psychological problems faced by an amputee are covered and succeeding chapters deal with phantom pain, after-care on discharge from hospital and the problems experienced with artificial limbs.

This is a valuable book, well illustrated and written clearly by an expert in amputee rehabilitation. I commend Mr Humm's *Rehabilitation of the Lower Limb Amputee* for its practical guidance. It will be found most useful by nurses, therapists and indeed doctors who have an interest in the problems of amputation.

*May 1977*                    A. E. S. RAINEY, MB, FRCSEd, FRCSI

# Preface

Progress in the rehabilitation of the lower limb amputee over the past years has been said to be slow but steady. This, however, refers mainly to the manufacture of a 'wonder limb' which it is hoped one day will replace adequately the human limb. With the exception of the members of the prosthetic team, the members of the total amputee rehabilitation team are not involved in the technical and engineering problems concerned in limb-making. The therapist and the nurse, however, are deeply involved in and are largely responsible for dealing with the equally important problems that arise in the course of preparing the amputee patient mentally and physically for limb wearing, and considerable progress has been made towards successfully overcoming these problems.

In this third edition much of Part One—which covers the pre-prosthetic phases of treatment, with the nurse and the therapist in a close working relationship and from which all patients benefit when team work is evident—has been rewritten. A new section has also been included which covers aspects of this specialized field of rehabilitation that will help towards a better understanding of the many problems involving the amputee patient. Some information on the bewildering 'phantom limb' has been included and the modern concept of amputee rehabilitation has been clearly set out. Some of the illustrations have been reproduced in the more modern setting of an amputee unit, and for the first time an index has been included to facilitate reference.

The therapist has been referred to generally as 'he' throughout the text but this reference is not intended to be discriminatory. It has been used for simplicity and clarity.

My sincere thanks are especially extended to Mr A. E. S. Rainey for reading the manuscript and writing the Foreword; also to Mr N. Backhouse, SRN, RCNT, Senior Nursing Tutor of the Wakefield School of Nursing and to Mr A. Willey, Head Remedial Gymnast, Staincliffe Hospital, Dewsbury, Yorkshire for their kindness and for the time devoted by them in helping me to prepare this third edition. Also to Hanger Ltd, Artificial Limb Makers, Roehampton, London, for illustrations.

*July 1977*                                              W. HUMM

# 1

# Introduction

The field of amputee rehabilitation has now become accepted as one among many specialized fields of physical rehabilitation. For those therapists wishing to specialize in this field it is necessary that they have a good understanding of the many requirements that involve the amputee patient. These requirements amount to a simple understanding of *why*, *how* and *when* the therapist should plan a correct and complete programme of physical treatment for each individual patient. It must be accepted, however, that the understanding of these requirements is not gained solely by qualification and registration as a member of any one remedial profession; it is achieved only by postgraduate study and experience in the fields of amputation surgery, nursing care, physical treatments, prosthetic requirements and, above all, in the acceptance of team work.

The author is not qualified to discuss amputation surgery but he can, however, discuss the levels of amputation best suited, under the heading of prosthetic requirements. The type of nursing care is vital for quick recovery of the amputee patient as well as the need for team work and good communication between the nurse and therapist. The requirement of the correct physical treatment plays a major role in obtaining the best possible end result. Such a result will not depend solely on a good stump and a good fitting limb; so much more will depend on the patient's physical treatment, which, if not continued in a progressive nature—particularly with an elderly amputee—could result in wasting the contribution from the other members of the health care team to the patient's rehabilitation.

On the question of prosthetic requirements, it would be fair to say that this is the essence of amputee rehabilitation. Without an understanding of this aspect, it could be said that the therapist and the nurse are practically working in the dark and unlikely to achieve the best possible end-result.

## THE MODERN CONCEPT

The modern concept of amputee rehabilitation is simply 'early re-habilitation'. This is best achieved by involving amputees, as soon as possible and in every possible way, in their own rehabilitation programmes. Every encouragement must be given to all patients to make them aware of what they themselves must do to enhance early rehabilitation. For example, they must not be allowed to wait until the nurse or the therapist comes into the ward to 'switch them on'. It is accepted, of course, that many patients in the beginning will need some individual assistance for a period of time; however, a working situation with one patient–one nurse or therapist must be recommended for a speedy introduction of the patient's personal independence in the ward and group therapy sessions in the amputee unit.

## THE TOTAL AMPUTEE REHABILITATION TEAM

The rehabilitation team could consist of twenty or more professional personnel who may become involved in the recovery of any one amputee patient. Of this large number, it is the therapist who is un-doubtedly the key worker in maintaining communication between all members of the team; without this vital link the therapist (with whom the patient will spend most of his or her time) will find progress at best delayed and at worst not going on at all.

A list of these members will invariably involve: the general practi-tioner; the surgeon and his surgical team; the ward sister and her nursing staff; the ward therapist and the unit therapist; the limb-fitting medical officer and his prosthetic team; the medical social worker; the community nurse; the hospital resettlement officer; and lastly the *patient*, who must at all times be considered the most impor-tant member of the team.

## THE ULTIMATE REMEDIAL AIM

The ultimate remedial aim is to assist and encourage each amputee who has been supplied with a prosthesis to become once again, or as near to, a normal member of the community, safe and independent on his or her prosthesis. For those amputee patients who are best advised (or prefer) to accept a wheelchair existence, then the same remedial aim is recommended.

### REASONS FOR AMPUTATION

The following information will indicate to the reader the various reasons for amputation and will show why the requirement of physical treatment for the large number of present day amputees is so vital.

It has been estimated that in the United Kingdom alone there are approximately 4500 new primary amputees each year. Of this figure the reasons for amputation are estimated as follows: 70% as a result of vascular disease; 10% as a result of other diseases; 17% because of trauma, road and industrial accidents, etc.; 3% because of congenital malformation during young adulthood or later years.

With such a high percentage of limbs lost because of vascular disease, it is not unreasonable to accept that most of these patients would be in the 60-plus age group, many of them presenting, on admission to hospital, a standard of physical fitness certainly below average and therefore requiring a carefully planned programme of physical treatment.

## LEVELS OF AMPUTATION

It is important that the nurse and the therapist are aware of the levels of amputation and their relationship to 'prosthetic requirements', particularly when faced with the problem of reassuring patients before or after amputation that all is not lost as to their future.

### THE SYME'S AMPUTATION

The Syme's amputation is often considered by the inexperienced to be a simple amputation of the foot, presenting little or no problems from the point of view of rehabilitation. Such an assumption is, however, a gross misconception and if careful consideration is not given to this level of amputation during the early phases of treatment by both the nurse and the therapist the patient's progress can be painfully retarded.

From the prosthetic point of view, the Syme's amputation was at one time considered unfavourable. It is, however, a satisfactory level of amputation for some patients, particularly for the young amputee where there is some epiphyseal development.

The therapist and the nurse need to understand some of the factors that help make it a successful limb-fitting level of amputation. There are two types of Syme's amputation; the classical Syme's as described by Syme and the modified Syme's. The former is an amputation through the ankle joint (disarticulation) and the latter is an amputation involving cutting through the tibia and fibula at approximately 2.5 cm above the level of the ankle joint. It is important, therefore, that the nurse and therapist should know which type of Syme's amputation they are treating or nursing, as there is a difference in the approach to weight-bearing exercises during the early postoperative treatment.

The classical Syme's presents a bulbous end stump covered with natural weight-bearing skin over the heel pad, which is placed over a wide area of *uncut bone*. With this type of amputation weight-bearing exercises and standing by the bed side can be safely started two weeks postoperatively, with care being taken not to displace the heel pad from its original position.

The modified Syme's presents *cut bone*, with a smaller weight-bearing area. The heel pad is covered with little or no natural weight-bearing skin. Here it is wiser to delay early weight-bearing until four to six weeks postoperatively, thus saving the patient unnecessary discomfort and avoiding the risk of moving the heel pad, as this is a big disadvantage to the fitting of a prosthesis. It is also very important for the exercises of weight-bearing to be progressed from partial to full weight-bearing very gently indeed, as full weight-bearing may never be achieved. Incorrect stump bandaging can also be the cause of moving the heel pad if it is not applied evenly around the distal end of the stump.

If the postoperative treatment of the Syme's amputee is taken too lightly—on the assumption that such a level of amputation would not present any problems—it may well delay the patient's progress because it could present a far greater problem for limb-fitting than would, for instance, a hip disarticulation.

A suggested approach to this problem is as follows. Ideally the stump should be placed in a plaster cast up to the tibial tuberosity immediately after amputation for a period of 10 to 14 days. Physical treatment during this time should consist of general exercises, specific quadriceps resisted exercises and crutch walking. The prevention of hip and knee flexion deformities is a primary aim at this stage of treatment. Following the removal of the plaster and the sutures, with the heel pad soundly fixed, progressive weight-bearing exercises could be started with care. In all instances of Syme's amputation, the patient should be referred to his nearest limb-fitting centre as soon as possible following the removal of the sutures.

### BELOW-KNEE AMPUTATION

This level of amputation can, undoubtedly, be considered as the best functional level. It provides two joints above the amputated stump thus enabling the patient to obtain good control of the prosthesis and a more natural walking gait with the below-knee patella tendon bearing limb (P.T.B.).

The ideal below-knee stump is one that measures 11.0–12.0 cm (4.5–5.0 in) from the medial condyle of the tibia to the distal end of the stump; the tip of the tibia is bevelled and covered by muscle tissue (myoplastic). However, in view of the advantages of retaining two joints and the P.T.B. limb, therapists could find themselves treating below-knee amputees with stumps shorter than 11.0 cm. In such cases great care must be taken to prevent knee flexion contractures, bearing in mind that the powerful hip extensor muscles are associated with knee flexion. It is necessary to point out, however, and important to remember that preference to full extension must be given to the hip joint.

### THROUGH-KNEE AMPUTATION (DISARTICULATION)

The through-knee amputation is one of disarticulation at the knee joint *with no cut bone*, thus providing the perfect end-bearing stump. Early weight-bearing and limb-fitting is possible with this level of amputation. The through-knee amputation has gained popularity over the past years in this country, particularly for the elderly patient. There are three important aspects of this level of amputation that the nurse and therapist should be aware so the benefit gained from the through-knee amputation is not lost.

The first of these is the prevention of hip flexion contractures. Surgically, hip flexion deformity is a contraindication for this level of amputation; this alone should be sufficient to remind therapists of its importance. However, in view of the long stump, 5° of flexion at the hip would be magnified at the distal end of stump, thus making limb-wearing difficult and incurring the loss of the natural end-bearing surface.

The second aspect is the ability to bear weight on the distal end of stump. This should be achieved as soon as possible in the physical treatment programme and it is suggested that this should start on the fifth or sixth day after amputation. The suture line is situated posteriorly and not affected when the patient—lying prone on the bed—attempts to press up into a kneeling position. This is then progressed until the patient is able to bear weight on a sorbo mattress. The lack of ability of these patients to bear weight early on the end of stump causes much delay during the later prosthetic phase of training.

The third aspect is the power of the abductor group of muscles working on the hip joint of the amputated side. Figure 22 (p. 79) shows the permanent prosthesis supplied to the through-knee amputee. It will be seen that no lateral support is given, as with the above-knee prosthesis (Fig. 20) where there is a pelvic band. The through-knee amputee, therefore, must provide his own lateral stability when using his limb. This can be made possible only if he is given the opportunity to build up his muscle power by specific resisted exercises; normal resisted exercises would have little or no effect on the sartorius, gluteus minimus and tensor fasciae latae muscles, which are all abductors that need to work statically, stabilizing the hip joint as the body weight passes over the joint.

Two other complications are seen from time to time during the rehabilitation of the through-knee amputee. These are a small localized area of skin necrosis over the condyle posteriorly and an effusion of synovial fluid under the skin flap. These will not necessarily cause suspension of treatment but they should be reported to the operating surgeon early and his decision must be final.

ABOVE-KNEE (MID-THIGH) AMPUTATION

It could be said that this is the most common level of amputation due mainly to the fact that it offers, in most cases, a better blood supply for both a healthy stump and an uneventful recovery. The ideal above-knee stump is one that measures about 25–30 cm (10–12 in) from the greater trochanter to the distal end of stump, having been amputated using the myoplastic technique. This particular stump provides both a good, strong functional action for controlling and management of the prosthesis and permits a good cosmetic finish.

Long stumps measuring more than 30 cm (12 in), which are recognized either as the long femoral stump or the Gritti–Stokes amputation presenting *cut bone* just above the level of the knee joint, will both present complications with regard to limb fitting. Because of the length of stump it is not possible to fit into the prosthesis a knee control unit without dropping the knee centre which results in an unsatisfactory cosmesis. A distance of 16 cm (6.5 in) is required below the distal end of stump for a good cosmetic fitting of a knee unit. To overcome this problem the long above-knee stumps are fitted with a modified above-knee limb with no knee control unit.

The nurse and the therapist when meeting the long femoral stump, or the Gritti–Stokes amputation (which are recognized by the absence of the femoral condyles) must become aware of the dangers of hip flexion contractures.

Short above-knee stumps measuring less than 20 cm would require a great deal more effort from the patient in the control and management of the above-knee prosthesis and may even result in the patient being unable to manage a free-knee mechanism. Once again the prevention of hip flexion contracture is of major importance.

## DISARTICULATION OF THE HIP

Disarticulation of the hip is self-explanatory. It might be pointed out that the reason for this level of amputation is not necessarily vascular disease, but also one of the other 10% of diseases, or major trauma. When the psychological problems for this patient have been overcome, the physical aspects of rehabilitation and limb wearing is not as difficult as one might assume.

## HEMIPELVECTOMY (HINDQUARTER AMPUTATION)

Hemipelvectomy is the highest level of amputation for the lower limb. The reasons for and all aspects of rehabilitation for the hindquarter amputee are the same as for the disarticulation of the hip.

## PHASES OF TREATMENT

In general terms, there are two phases of treatment, firstly the pre-prosthetic phase and, secondly, the prosthetic phase. However, to ensure the best programme of amputee rehabilitation, four phases of treatment are recommended and these are discussed more fully under their individual headings in the following chapters.

### PROSTHETIC REQUIREMENTS

The understanding of the prosthetic requirements is the essence of planning a correct programme of amputee rehabilitation. The nurse and the therapist must have an appreciation of the following requirements related to the prosthesis:

1. Levels of amputation and their appropriate prostheses
2. Correct application of a prosthesis
3. What constitutes a correct fitting socket, with particular reference to the weight-bearing area
4. The reasons for variations in size of stumps
5. The importance of correct stump bandaging
6. The association of body mechanics with engineering
7. The different types of prosthetic mechanism (locks and suspensions etc.)
8. The importance of correct standing balance and transfer of body-weight
9. That re-education of walking alone is not prosthetic training
10. All possible functional activities should be taught
11. Prosthetic training has no time factor; it should continue until the ultimate remedial aim has been achieved
12. The therapist considering whether the prosthesis is going to be an asset or a hindrance for the patient's future

### PROSTHETIC REQUIREMENTS OF THE PATIENT

The understanding of the above prosthetic requirements by the therapist will indicate why the patient must be encouraged to achieve the following to become a successful limb wearer.

1. The will-power to succeed
2. Maximum physical fitness
3. Prevention of joint contractures

4. Mobile joints above the level of amputation
5. Healthy functional stump
6. Hardening of the ischial seating area
7. Confident free standing balance on the sound leg
8. Strong quadriceps on the amputated side of the below-knee and through-knee amputee
9. Strong abductor power of the hip on the amputated side of the below-knee and through-knee amputee
10. Good extension and adduction of the hip on the amputated side for the above-knee amputee
11. Strong upper limbs, particularly for the bilateral amputee
12. The patient's understanding of stump care and limb management

THE AMPUTEE UNIT

The best results for amputee rehabilitation are gained when patients are treated in a *group* with other amputees in various phases of treatment, and not individually or with other patients with different conditions being treated in walking classes. It is recommended that in hospitals or rehabilitation centres, where amputees are being treated, a specific section should be set aside or converted into an amputee unit which requires no extra staff, space or special equipment other than that found in any normal remedial gymnasium or activity area. Such a unit could be developed in a space measuring approximately 8 m × 13 m with the following equipment: two sets of firm walking rails; exercise mats; single step and ramp; set of stairs; small strip of carpet; medicine balls (20 kg); light plastic balls; exercise sticks; weight and weight bags; springs.

Only one golden rule should be observed: the unit at all times should be under the strict and sole supervision of the same experienced therapist.

A suggested time factor for patients attending the unit are as follows: all *in-patients* should attend daily for not less than one hour per period, this being followed by a further period of exercises in the ward. *Out-patients*, with or without limbs, should attend for two-hourly periods three times a week (Monday, Wednesday and Friday) or four-hourly periods, twice weekly. The amputee patient should attend continuously until either the ultimate remedial aim has been achieved or it has been decided that the patient will not remain safe on a prosthesis and limb wearing is postponed or cancelled.

The general practice of treating the amputee patient for short periods twice or three times a week for a set period of attendances, and possibly being seen by a different therapist during this time, is most unsuitable and unlikely to lead to the best possible result. Most elderly patients, in particular, take time to fully understand the instructions given and become confused if these differ slightly from one therapist to another.

# Part One

# Early and Intermediate Phases
## (Pre-prosthetic)

# 2

# The Nurse

Experience has shown that in many hospitals a gap exists between the work of the nursing staff and the therapist. This applies to almost every form of physical treatment administered in the wards. The need for members of the physical medicine department to work in the wards should offer an excellent opportunity for the therapist and nurse to join forces and work together as a team, and consciously acknowledge the importance of this in hastening the patient's recovery.

The nurse must be considered a vital member of any rehabilitation team and should be encouraged to take part in this work. Nurses are trained to be observant of their patients' needs at all times, and are undoubtedly in the position to maintain continuity of treatment throughout the day.

From the therapist's point of view, there are many factors to be observed during his absence from the ward. It would also be a great asset to the patient if the nurse were aware of all important aspects of rehabilitation. Of course it is not suggested that the nurse should take on the role of the therapist or even carry out this work if a therapist is available, but there are a number of occasions when the patient would benefit from the nurse who knows *why* and *how* to follow the programme of physical treatment.

The nurse should be aware of two most important factors: the correct bed and chair posture, by the amputee, as a preventive measure against flexion contracture of hip and knee joints; the specific method of stump bandaging for early limb fitting and, in particular, the reasons for it. It would be wrong to assume that the nurse cannot do the stump bandage. However, methods do vary a little in the limb service training as well as in nurse training schools.

Apart from the recent amputee who requires a stump bandage, many established limb wearers are admitted into hospital for reasons other than their amputation. Although the cause of admission is adequately dealt with, care of the amputation stump is often overlooked. Should this happen and the stump not be bandaged correctly, it may cause unnecessary delay in limb fitting. The nurse may meet some opposition from her patient who will state that he has not bandaged his stump for many years, with no ill effect. This may well be true, but prevention is better than cure, and when the nurse is aware that her patient may not wear his limb for any length of time, she should explain the need for stump bandaging, and gently insist on its being done.

Some patients who have been confined to bed even for a few days and have not bandaged their stumps have complained later that the stump had swollen and made limb wearing difficult. This is a common cause of stump damage; the stump becomes too large to fit the socket, which causes some constriction of the circulation, and epidermoid cysts form in the region of the groin and are difficult to clear up if the socket is a tight fit. Similar changes may take place in hospital patients and illness or surgery is likely to alter normal metabolism and so affect the stump. Correct stump bandaging will help to avoid these problems.

The prevention of flexion contracture of the hip and knee joints is equally important for the established limb wearer who is to be subjected to long periods of non-limb wearing as it is for the primary amputee. Correct bed posture and sitting posture are of vital importance. The nurse needs to be alert for the above-knee amputee who is constantly curled up on his bed, or sitting in his wheelchair for long periods with his stump, or stumps, in an abducted position. Below-knee amputees tend to favour sitting with the amputated limb crossed over the sound knee. These are bad habits and detrimental to future limb wearing. A simple counteraction to this is to encourage the patient to take the 'prone lying' position on his bed for periods of not less than thirty minutes.

Fracture boards play an important part in the prevention of flexion contractures and should be accepted as an essential part of the amputee's bed. Contraindications arise occasionally and permission for the use of boards should first be obtained from the surgeon or physician in charge of the patient. Orthopaedic wards are normally well equipped with boards but general wards may not be, and as a result many amputee patients spend a deal of time in bed without them. The nurse might be the first to notice that boards were not being used and could ask her ward sister if they may be used. However, the prime responsibility would be with the therapist if he were involved with that patient's care.

There are many occasions when the nurse can assist her patient, particularly the elderly patient, with the application of his limb. It is, then, necessary for her to understand the various techniques used if she is to be successful. Incorrect application of a prosthesis can quickly bring about stump damage.

The nurse will very probably not have received specific training on this point, and so she must look to the therapist for encouragement and guidance; obviously, the right place to impart this information is in the ward where the therapist can be seen at work. The ward sister is in charge there and responsible for the coordination of the patients' treatment and for the work and training of her nurses. If a suitable approach is made by the therapist, most ward sisters would welcome the opportunity for their nurses to learn the appropriate techniques.

In many hospitals, nursing homes and clinics the therapist is an occasional visitor only and the duration of each visit is inevitably limited. In such situations the nurse can be a great asset to the patient if she has some knowledge and interest in the programme of rehabilitating the lower limb amputee.

# 3

# Psychological Problems

Patients admitted to hospital with some vascular or traumatic condition of the lower limb, which may necessitate amputation, are often in the ward for a day or so pending a final decision by the surgeon to operate. This short period is a blessing for the therapist; it gives him the opportunity to assess the patient and to decide how best to reassure him that, should amputation be necessary, all will not be lost. He should also explain to the patient that, by cooperating and working together, they will achieve a very considerable degree of mobility and comfort for him.

Some patients will be so pain-sickened that they will be glad to rid themselves of the cause and settle for a wheelchair. These are the most difficult patients to cope with. Others are so afraid that they will never walk again that they are, consequently, very loath to accept the surgeon's advice for surgical intervention. This category generally embraces the older type of patient. There is also the younger family man who feels that the absence of a limb will prevent him providing for, or adequately looking after, his family; to him the world has come to an end.

The state of mind of these patients is critical; some may show it openly, others may not. Nevertheless, every effort must be made to encourage them and to assure them that a great deal can be achieved.

How, then, is this problem to be tackled? Firstly, the patient must be able to accept the therapist as a friend whom he can trust. This, of course, is common sense, and no therapist should need reminding of the necessity of gaining such confidence. Secondly, it is necessary to convince the patient that he has no doubt passed many amputees in the streets walking so well that he has never noticed their disability; he must be convinced that it is not difficult to manage an artificial limb with the correct techniques of prosthetic training. Finally, if through the loss of a limb the patient is unable to return to his previous work, he must be made aware that there are many suitable training centres under the control of the Employment Services Agency Scheme, where a new trade or profession can be taught.

There must, of course, be some necessary adjustment to the normal routines of life but this is seldom sufficient to be unbearable. The extent of such an adjustment cannot be truly assessed until the patient has had an opportunity of using his artificial limb. However, the therapist who can set the patient's mind at rest has taken the first step towards success inasmuch as the latter is ready to accept the fact that he is about to become an amputee.

MENTAL AND PHYSICAL ASSESSMENT

The need for an early mental and physical assessment of the patient's possible potential as a limb wearer is vital to all members of the total rehabilitation team. It is, therefore, beneficial if during this early meeting with the patient the therapist makes a provisional assessment.

For the experienced therapist in this field it should not require the expertise of a psychologist to determine whether the patient has the mental capacity to follow simple rules of safety instructions in the management of wearing a prosthesis. From the physical aspect the following points should be noted and recorded: the patient's age; general medical condition (obtained from the nursing staff); body weight, i.e. obese, heavy, medium, light, frail; past period of inactivity; ranges of movement of all limbs and trunk; muscle power—particularly the extensors of hip and knee joints; any joint contractures or deformities; any other complication such as poor sight, hearing, etc.

These factors should be recorded and filed, if there is any doubt as to whether the patient may not be suitable for limb wearing. Such information can be most helpful to the operating surgeon and the medical social worker, and can save so much time in the future planning of the patient's welfare.

# 4

# Pre-prosthetic
# Physical Treatment

It cannot be emphasized too strongly that the end result gained by amputees on their prostheses is not due solely to the level of amputation or the type of limb they are wearing, but is determined by the standard of physical fitness of each patient at the beginning of the later, prosthetic phase of treatment. To achieve the best result three factors are essential:

1. The patient's will-power to succeed
2. The therapist's knowledge of the patient's physical and prosthetic requirements
3. The time and space to achieve these requirements

## PHASE ONE: PREOPERATIVE TREATMENT

Preoperative exercise therapy is not an innovation in the programme of amputee rehabilitation but it is becoming more popular and necessary. Unfortunately, some therapists and medical officers appear to be unaware of the real benefits gained from even short periods of preoperative physical treatment. It may well mean treating a patient who has a painful leg, a gangrenous foot or varicose ulcers but, nevertheless, much progress can be made towards preparing the patient for limb-wearing.

Two essential factors are gained from preoperative treatment. Firstly, physical preparation is started early and the pre-proceptive impulses of balance on two legs are maintained up to the very last moment before amputation (this is most vital for speedy progress on a prosthesis) and, secondly, it is an excellent time for making a

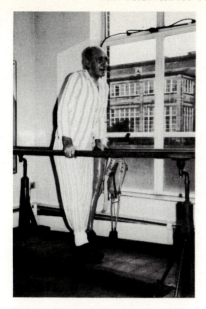

Fig. 1. Preoperative, partial weight-bearing walking in stocking feet. Gangrenous foot padded and bandaged, three days before amputation.

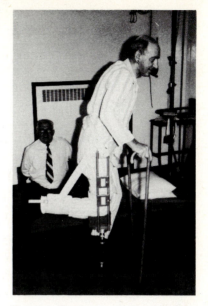

Fig. 2. The preoperative kneeling prosthesis, two days before amputation. Note weakness of left leg due to long periods of inactivity at home. The patient in the background is a bilateral above-knee amputee preparing for walking exercises before limb-wearing, as shown in Fig. 18.

start on the patient's mental rehabilitation by allowing him or her to meet and see other amputees at various stages of training; this is linked with a simple explanation of the importance of exercise before amputation and the reassurance that all is not lost.

A suggested period of preoperative treatment is one to five days, depending on the urgency of amputation. Short but frequent periods of free exercises given in all possible starting positions to mobilize joints and stimulate the circulation. If the affected limb cannot be moved actively it should be placed in an overhead sling suspension, the point of suspension being directly over the hip joint (this being the most important joint—whether the intended site of amputation is to be below, through or above the knee joint).

Single leg standing balance (sound leg) and short periods of walking between the walking rails are of tremendous value. A gangrenous foot can be adequately padded and bandaged to allow the patient to make an early start, using the rails for partial weight-bearing (Fig. 1). In some instances it may be necessary to ask if analgesics can be given, perhaps half an hour before treatment starts, to help ease the pain so that physical treatment can be given.

A great deal more time and benefit is gained by teaching crutch walking during this early treatment period. One can well imagine the apprehension of any patient who is required to use crutches for the first time just a few days following amputation. The use of a temporary preoperative kneeling appliance (Fig. 2) fitted to the affected limb is a further means of enhancing the patient's progress. It is recommended that, when this phase of treatment is not requested, the therapist should then suggest to the surgeon that periods of pre-operative physical treatments are vitally important to the amputee's future progress on his or her prosthesis.

All treatments preoperatively should be carried out, wherever possible, in the amputee unit. If physical treatment is not allowed at this stage, it is still psychologically beneficial if the patient can meet other amputees in the unit on a social basis.

It is, of course, understood that the ultimate degree of fitness will be determined by the type of patient with whom the therapist is involved. Such cases as cardiac failure, arthritis, muscular paresis, etc. must all be taken into consideration, but even these patients must still achieve the maximum amount of their physical exercise tolerance.

## PHASE TWO: THE IMMEDIATE POSTOPERATIVE PHASE IN THE WARD

The immediate postoperative phase of treatment concerns the ward nurse and the ward therapist: the therapist will acknowledge that he is not able to observe the patient as frequently as the nurse and therefore, a close working relationship during this phase is vital. The patient must be aware of this joint effort so as to avoid any reluctance to follow the nurse's instructions with regard to physical treatment which may have been requested by the therapist. However, before stressing any physical treatment, it would be beneficial to point out the importance of several aspects of nursing care, which, if not observed, could well retard the patient's physical progress.

## BED POSTURE

It has been pointed out that most lower limb amputees are likely to be of the over-60 age group and not in a good condition of general fitness. This may mean an inability to move about the bed at will and if these patients are left lying for too long in one position, joint stiffness, joint contractures and pressure sores are inevitable. To help prevent these complications arising the following advice is given: place fracture boards under the mattress thus providing a firm base which helps the patient to move more easily on the bed (the fracture boards also adds greatly to the prevention of hip flexion contractures); encourage the patient to lie flat in the supine position, with the stump relaxed and resting on the mattress. This position of bed posture permits easier movement of most other joints. Movement of the stump by the patient in this position is also much easier if the bottom sheet is checked to see that it has not wrinkled up and causing some resistance to the stump, through the bandage or dressing, when attempting to slide the stump from the position of abduction to adduction. Patients who are left lying supine with their stumps in an abducted position for long periods are subjected to a possible abduction contracture. It is important, therefore, that each patient is able to move the stump freely in bed. Most amputees, once able to turn onto their sound side, will do so and will flex the hip of the amputated side for the purpose of supporting the stump with their hands as a means of comfort. This is a most natural situation but it must be discouraged if a hip flexion deformity is to be prevented. It will be observed also, that almost every amputee finds the position of side-lying the best for sleeping. It is recommended that the nurse, when waking the patient each morning, should advise him or her to adopt the supine position, thus allowing the stump to rest flat on the mattress, and explaining the importance of this position in preventing hip flexion contractures.

## STUMP INFECTION

Stump infection is not unknown to cause a delaying of early rehabilitation and the most common cause is due to infection from urine.

Some elderly patients become a little incontinent and dribble unknowingly or are unable to use a urine bottle correctly and this makes the dressing become wet and the stump infected; the nurse and the therapist are strongly advised to inform the ward sister should there be any question of this happening. An immediate application of a new bandage or dressing could save a long delay in the programme of rehabilitation and prevent much discomfort for the patient.

## PHYSICAL TREATMENT

### FIRST THREE DAYS: POSTOPERATIVE CHEST THERAPY

Amputee patients of all levels of amputation should, for the *first three days*, be given the normal procedure of postoperative chest therapy. Those patients with a chest complication will of course require this treatment more specifically for longer periods.

### FOURTH POSTOPERATIVE DAY

Gentle *assisted active movements* of the stump—mainly *adduction* and *extension* for the above-knee amputee—should be given; *extension* and *abduction* of the hip and *extension* of the knee for the below-knee amputee; *extension* and *abduction* of the hip for the through-knee amputee. All these assisted active movements should be given two or three times daily for periods lasting no longer than 15 minutes. The importance of the patient being able to perform these movements actively, and as early as possible, must be stressed. The therapist, however, must be aware of the over-enthusiastic patient trying to perform active stump movements too soon, as this could result in producing a more painful stump than might be expected from this early postoperative stage.

   Between the periods of assisted movements of the stump, the patient must be encouraged to carry out general, active movements of the sound leg, arms and trunk. The exercise therapy approach for the Syme's amputee will be as for the below-knee. The early physical treatment for the hip disarticulation and the hindquarter amputee will consist of general exercises only to the sound leg, arms and trunk until the sixth postoperative day.

SIXTH POSTOPERATIVE DAY

From this time onward and until the sutures have been removed, stump exercises should progress both to more free active exercises, and to early resisted exercises. Progressive resisted exercises to the sound leg and arms should be encouraged. If allowed out of the ward, a social visit to the amputee unit is always beneficial. For the hip disarticulation and the hindquarter amputees, these patients should now start gentle static contractions of the abdominal and glutei muscle groups, followed by small-range rotation and side flexion of the trunk which should be progressed accordingly.

TENTH POSTOPERATIVE DAY

According to the patient's general condition, all levels of amputation should be treated in the amputee unit as *phase three* of the rehabilitation programme following the tenth postoperative day.

SITTING OUT

Many ward sisters and surgeons like to see their amputee patients sitting out as early as possible. With some patients this could be on the second or third postoperative day. There must be no objections to this forward thinking provided that the following factors are observed and understood.

Lower limb amputees who are allowed to sit out for longer than two hours in a low, soft-seated armchair, sitting on pillows or air rings, comfortable and undemanding will ultimately find limb wearing difficult and this will delay early rehabilitation. This particular type of chair, being low and soft, will encourage hip and knee flexion contractures and will inhibit free movement of the stump, sound leg, and trunk (Fig. 3). The soft seat will not help in the important aspect of hardening of the ischial seating area (ischial tuberosities) upon which the amputee will be full weight-bearing when using his or her temporary pylon. To obtain the best possible results from the sitting out period, the following system is suggested: two hours sitting in a comfortable chair; two hours sitting on a hard-seated chair with a straight back, with the chair facing the bed thus providing a suitable surface for the patient's reading matter and food tray etc. (Fig. 4). The discomfort from the hard seat will encourage the patient to support himself by his hands on the bed and raise himself up onto

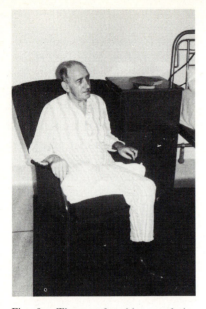

Fig. 3. The comfortable armchair, four days after amputation. Note the position of the above-knee stump.

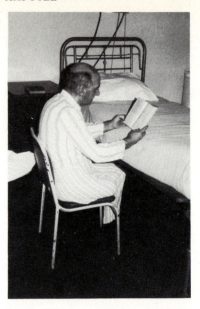

Fig. 4. The firm seated straight-back chair. Note good position of the stump and lumbar spine, also patient's mental state settled to concentrated reading four days after amputation.

the sound leg thus providing active exercise for the sound leg, arms and trunk. In the very early days, this activity will probably require the attention of the nurse or the therapist until the patient becomes more confident.

Following a period of sitting on the hard-seat chair, the patient should be encouraged to lie supine on the bed and to continue with the programme of bed exercises shown by the therapist. It is acknowledged that in these early days, sitting for long periods will not be possible with some patients and they should, therefore, be allowed only short periods of sitting in a soft, comfortable armchair and then be permitted to lie on top of the bed.

CRUTCH WALKING IN THE WARD

Whether the amputee patient has been taught the techniques of crutch walking preoperatively or not, it must be accepted that the patient will be very apprehensive when asked to do this a few days following amputation; the fear of falling and knocking the stump will be foremost in his or her mind. It is not uncommon, therefore, to find that the patient is holding the stump forward in a position of hip flexion which encourages a hip contracture and produces a poor sense of balance on the sound leg. If the patient is unable to coordinate the stump with the crutches, he or she should be encouraged to let the stump hang loosely, taking short steps as a swing-through action is carried out by the sound leg, the body-weight being taken on the arms through the crutches.

WALKING FRAMES

The use of walking frames encourages the amputee patient to hop on the sound leg and is not recommended. There is considerable danger of the patient falling backwards and more important, an unjustifiable stress is put on to the sound leg. It must be remembered that if the cause of amputation was vascular disease, the disease will not have been cured by the amputation and the sound leg may itself be suspect.

Following the removal of all sutures, and with the sound healing of the stump, firm stump bandaging should be started in order to condition the stump for limb wearing (see Chapter 8, Stump Bandaging).

BILATERAL AMPUTEES

Bilateral amputations are seldom ever done at the same time, so the immediate postoperative physical treatment will be the same for each level of amputation as it takes place.

The postoperative physical treatment for the bilateral amputee calls for a considerable amount of thought and appreciation of the physical requirements for managing two artificial limbs. It would be wrong to assume, for instance, that it can only be twice as difficult as dealing with the single amputee; the physical and mental effort needed are increased far more. Bearing this in mind and also the age group involved, the various causes of amputation and their relationship to physical effort, the therapist will clearly see the difficulties that lie ahead, not only for the patient but for all members of the rehabilitation team whose task it is to restore the patient to a state of personal independence and safety. The following is a suggested plan of how this problem might be overcome.

A meeting of the rehabilitation team should be held to discuss whether the patient is a suitable candidate for artificial limbs or whether he or she should be trained for a wheelchair existence. There are many times when this becomes a difficult decision to make. Nevertheless, where there is the slightest element of doubt the benefit should be given to the patient and it may well be that the patient will not make much progress on artificial limbs, yet benefit from the use of temporary rocker pegs even if only to be able to stand from his wheelchair. Many functions are easier to manage for those looking after the patient at home if the patient is able to stand.

The answer to this is generally found by examining the patient's general medical condition, age group and the result of a physical and mental assessment, plus the advantage artificial limbs would be to the patient at home and in improving their social life. Should it be decided that the patient should have artificial limbs, an early appointment should be made for him or her to attend the nearest limb-fitting centre. From then on a programme of progressive physical treatment must be started and continued until the delivery of a pair of temporary rocker pegs. Whatever the level of the bilateral site of amputation, the stumps should be treated as previously stated. Other considerations of importance include the points that all bilateral below-knee amputees must have a period of concentrated work on the quadriceps muscles and that the patient should spend some time every day balancing and walking on the knees as soon as the condition of the stumps permits. It is also highly important to watch for any flexion contractures of the hip joint; good sound below-knee stumps with full extension of the knees are wasted if there is evidence of hip flexion contracture. The hip abductor group of muscles must also be given strong resisted exercises to provide sound lateral stability when walking on the prostheses. The upper limbs and shoulder girdle muscle groups should be developed to a state of hypertrophy if possible. This is vitally important for all levels of bilateral amputees, since without strong upper limbs the ability to negotiate steps and stairs and to sit and stand from a chair is difficult and unsafe.

For the bilateral above-knee amputees it is necessary that they are given the opportunity of taking a little weight on the end of their stumps, by lying prone on a sorbo mattress and introducing press-up exercises. This was, at one time, a difficult but most beneficial stump exercise for the patient to perform, although it is now more acceptable and possible since the introduction of the myoplastic surgical technique, whereby muscles are sutured over the end of the cut bone. To help harden the ischial seating area for full weight-bearing on the rocker pegs, these patients should be encouraged to bounce themselves up and down on the unit floor. Group activities and group recreational therapy periods with the bilateral amputee sitting on the floor (prostheses off) are most beneficial if the bilateral amputee is to become a successful limb wearer.

## PHASE THREE: IN THE AMPUTEE UNIT

Patients attending the amputee unit for the treatment of phase three (pre-prosthetic training), would be (1) those in-patients being seen preoperatively or those waiting discharge from the ward following amputation and who are attending the unit daily; (2) those patients who are at home but waiting to be called to the limb-fitting centre and attending the unit as out-patients three times weekly for periods not less than two hours for each visit.

The following is a suggested programme of physical treatment for all levels of amputation postoperatively and waiting delivery of their first temporary pylon: free-standing balance on the sound leg, followed by exercise of hip up-drawing of the amputated side, ensures that the stump is being held in good alignment and is not held in an abducted position; continued specific exercises of the stump followed by resisted exercises are recommended which would include kneeling balance and activities in kneeling for the below-knee amputees; end-bearing balance for the through-knee amputees; hardening of the ischial seating area for all amputees; general and specific exercises to the upper limbs, trunk and sound leg by means of group and recreational therapy. In addition to helping build up muscle power, recreational group therapy helps to break down the boredom of exercise and stimulates an atmosphere of competitive spirit (it would be wrong to assume that the elderly patient does not enjoy playing minor games: if the unit atmosphere is right and the therapist's enthusiasm is evident, the elderly amputee will enjoy every moment of recreational therapy, particularly if he or she is involved with patients with similar disabilities).

## GROUP DISCUSSIONS

Small group discussions are of great value to the amputee, as they embrace instructions and advice covering the 'aids to daily living' which are essential for those amputees who live alone or use wheelchairs in the house. Instructions and advice in stump bandaging should be given to the patient, relatives and other interested personnel—including hospital and community nurses—all of whom find themselves involved with the rehabilitation of the amputee. Small group discussions between those amputees with fitted limbs and those without limbs will be found most helpful and perhaps best achieved during a coffee- or tea-break.

It is here in the amputee unit that the nurse and the therapist will see the result and gain satisfaction from their work and encouragement of guiding the amputee patient through the first half of the total physical rehabilitation programme.

Many amputees have been deprived of making full use of their artificial limbs because of simple physical failure and lack of understanding. It is during the pre-prosthetic phases of treatment in the ward and in the amputee unit, where amputees can meet and work together, that they become able to accept their disabilities more readily and are prepared to take the next step forward to becoming successful limb wearers.

It is no exaggeration to say that there have been cases of unilateral amputees arriving at the limb fitting centre to take delivery of their temporary pylon unable to stand on the so-called good leg, the quadriceps muscles of which are so poor that they prevent them doing so; likewise, there have been bilateral amputees who have been unable to take off their jackets, the reason being lack of general mobilization of the shoulder girdle and long periods of inactivity sitting at home, perhaps just waiting for someone to advise them. Bearing these facts in mind, it must be clearly seen and understood by the ward and unit therapists that their responsibility does not end when the stump is soundly healed.

# 5

# The Phantom Limb

Many lower limb amputees will, at some time following amputation, complain or comment on experiencing the 'phantom limb'. As such, there is very little the nurse and the therapist can do about this situation, other than to explain to the patient that it is a normal aftermath of amputation, and that as the phantom limb becomes associated with the artificial limb the patient will quickly learn to ignore this strange experience.

## THE PAINFUL PHANTOM LIMB

Fewer patients complain of the painful phantom limb but, when they do, the nurse and the therapist must show concern, for although it would be very easy to say that an absent limb could not possibly be painful, the patient knows differently. This phenomemon could be related to the memory bank of the brain, and the patient, having suffered much pain prior to amputation, is on occasion reminded of this. It would appear that the memory has not, as yet, become orientated to the absence of the painful limb; fortunately, this orientation occurs and the painful phantom limb tends to disappear (a feature of the magical 'mind').

It must be remembered, however, that some patients will complain of the phantom limb being painful, but mistaking this for the painful stump. The therapist should, therefore, try to identify which is the true cause of pain. If the patient is asked to point to the area of pain, he or she will indicate an area *below* the level of the amputation, normally this is down at the foot. This indication could be accepted as a painful phantom, and the above explanation could be given to the patient with confidence. On the other hand, however, should the patient indicate the distal end of stump or thereabouts as the painful area, then this should be accepted as a *painful stump* (not phantom pain) and reported to the operating surgeon. Such painful stumps are due to neuroma, neuritis, sciatica, adhesions, or sepsis and should be reported early. If the condition does not settle following a course of injections then surgical intervention may be necessary.

### PHANTOM LIMB TREATMENTS (PHYSICAL)

Throughout the years, several types of remedial treatments have been tried to ease the symptoms of the phantom limb; percussion, ice therapy, deep massage, tight bandaging and short-wave diathermy have all been used but with no sufficient evidence to claim a complete cure. Such treatments are no longer recommended.

In view of the advanced surgical techniques of amputation surgery, the painful stump is seldom seen these days. Should the therapist be faced with this problem with a present day amputee, it would be advisable to include in his investigation a check on the patient's posture when standing and sitting with and without the prosthesis on and, perhaps, suggest a radiograph to be taken of the lumbar spine to ensure that the painful stump is not due to bad posture or referred pain from a low back disorder.

It is important to know and remember that many of the elderly amputees, particularly the bilateral amputee when wearing artificial limbs, will complain of low back pain. Much of this is due to muscular strain in maintaining an upright posture for correct posture and balance on their limbs. Fortunately, this tends to settle fairly quickly and, if not, it may be found that the patient is suffering some osteoarthritis of the lumbar spine.

# 6

# Discharge from Hospital

At the time of discharge, most patients will have had some three to six weeks in hospital, during which time they may or may not have been fully occupied in the rehabilitation department.

Whether or not these patients have been fully occupied in hospital, they nearly all tend to sit at home and do nothing. Little do they appreciate that this can be a critical period in their rehabilitation. It is then up to the therapist to ensure that his previous efforts to maintain a reasonable standard of the patient's general fitness are not wasted. This standard can be achieved only by the continuous repetition of the patients doing almost everything for themselves. They must know how and why they bandage their stumps; also, how and why they must remain active at home.

The time elapsing between patients leaving hospital and receiving their first temporary pylon can vary between four and eight weeks; during this time they will have attended the limb centre for examination and to be measured for their first socket.

So often, on delivery of the primary prosthesis, it is found that the stump has increased in size or a contracture has become evident. The result is (1) a new socket may be necessary, (2) an adjustment to the socket is required, or (3) it may be thought that prosthetic training will reduce the stump to its original state. Whatever the medical officer in charge decides, it is certain that the patient's progress will be delayed. Every effort must be made, therefore, to see that the patient is well-briefed on stump bandaging and on the type of exercises he should continue to do at home following discharge from hospital.

The community nurse and members of the voluntary medical services are often called upon to visit the amputee in his home. This visit may be at the request of the patient's hospital, his general practitioner, or the patient himself and the purpose could be for one of many reasons. Because the patient is an amputee the home visitor might well be faced with questions which she may be a little apprehensive about answering correctly. To help all those concerned, a number of the most likely questions and answers are listed below.

Following a request to visit such a patient the visitor should first try to find out whether the patient has just returned home from hospital following his amputation, or whether he has his artificial limb and has had some instruction on how to use it. This information will help the home visitor and prevent many problems from arising for, if a patient has not yet been seen and registered at his nearest limb-fitting centre, any questions that concern his artificial limb cannot be answered adequately by the home visitor.

The following questions and answers are a selection that might be expected from the amputee who has just returned home from hospital, and has not yet received his artificial limb.

*Can you bandage my stump?*

Yes. Then follow the instructions on stump bandaging shown on pp. 44–7. The inexperienced will no doubt find that applying a stump bandage for the first time can be a little difficult. Do not be alarmed; this is quite common. Only by constant practice can one become expert at this. To understand the aims and purpose of stump bandaging is more important than the various methods of application. It should be remembered, however, that it is better not to bandage the stump at all than to bandage it badly.

*How often should my stump be bandaged?*

At this stage the stump should remain bandaged day and night, the bandage being taken off only when washing or exercising the stump. This is the general practice for all amputees. However, should there be any doubt as to whether the stump should be left unbandaged, consult the patient's medical officer.

*Can you supply me with another bandage?*
Yes, if it is the correct size and type of bandage as given on p. 43. If not, then the patient must apply to the physical medicine department at his hospital.

*Can you attend to the dressing of the wound on my stump?*
Yes, but first receive instructions from the patient's medical officer. Keep the dressing as small as possible and continue with stump bandaging unless instructed not to do so by the hospital or the patient's medical officer.

*I can still feel the toes and the foot that were amputated. Is this all right, or is it my imagination?*
This is known as the phantom limb and is experienced by most amputees at some time or other. It can sometimes be a painful 'phantom limb', and in such cases the patient should report it to his medical officer. Amputees who experience a painless 'phantom limb' very soon learn to live with it, particularly when they are wearing their artificial limb (see Chapter 5).

*For how long must I continue with the fracture boards under my mattress?*
If the patient is elderly and has both legs amputated, and needs to spend long periods in bed, then the fracture boards must be used at all times. On the other hand if the patient is not old, has only one leg amputated and is active out of bed, then a firm mattress would suffice. The object and purpose of using fracture boards under the mattress are to help in the prevention of hip flexion contracture, and to enable the patient to move about the bed easily by providing a firm base.

*Can I have a bath?*
Yes, this is most important. The amputee should bath at least twice a week unless there are some contraindications for not doing so.

*How do I get into the bath with only one leg?*
This is easier than one would think, but so much depends on the age and general physical condition of the patient. For those who are able, the following procedure should be carried out. Place a large

bath towel or a non-skid rubber mat in the bath and run the water to approximately 25 cm (10 in) at the desired temperature. A small wooden stool is put into the bath. The patient sits on a chair beside the bath, he undresses, turns towards the bath placing the sound leg into the bath. He now takes hold of the bath sides, or a small fitted rail fixed to the wall, and lowers himself down on to the wooden stool and then into the bath. A little assistance may be needed at the first few attempts until the patient has gained self-confidence. To get out of the bath, he first sits up on the stool and runs out the water; while this is happening the top half of his body can be dried.

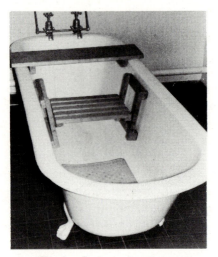

Fig. 5.   Bath stool and seat.

By reversing the method of sitting down, the patient can now stand up and sit on the bath side, and then move on to the chair. The lower half of the body can now be dried in safety.

Most single amputees will manage this quite well after a few attempts. The home visitor must be quite certain before she encourages the patient into the bath that his sound leg and arms are good and strong. Any attempt at lifting the amputee out of the bath is dangerous for both patient and home visitor.

For the amputee who has lost both legs the process is of course more difficult, but not impossible. Where such circumstances arise the home visitor should consult the physical medicine department of the patient's hospital for advice and guidance, as it is just as important for the bilateral amputee to know how to get into and out of a bath at home. Fig. 5 shows a most useful bathroom twin-set for the amputee, in particular for one with both legs amputated. The set can be purchased ready-made, but could easily be improvised by a handyman. The patient would move from his chair on to the wooden seat placed across the bath, then on to the stool, and from the stool into the bath. To get out of the bath the methods of getting into the bath would be repeated, but in reverse. It will be obvious, however, that the patient must have strong upper limbs to be able to lower and lift himself in and out of the bath with safety.

*Now that I have lost both my legs how do I manage the toilet?*

The first consideration here must be where the toilet is situated. If it is convenient and on the same level with no steps or stairs to negotiate, and the patient can wheel his wheelchair through the door space up to the toilet seat, there is little difficulty in moving off the chair seat on to the toilet. This can be made much easier if rails can be fitted each side of the toilet. Where, for no matter what reason, it is not possible to get the wheelchair up to the toilet seat there is little that the home visitor can do other than suggest the use of a commode until such time as the patient receives his artificial legs. In most cases where this problem arises, it will be found that the hospital medical social worker will doubtless have had it in hand.

*Can you lift me from my bed into my wheelchair?*

No, it is dangerous to lift or carry amputees. Two methods can be used. If the wheelchair has removable arm rests, remove one side and place the chair sideways to the bed, and encourage the patient to move off the bed into the chair. This form of activity is very important to the patient's future. If the arm rests are not removable, place the chair facing the bed, wheel brakes on. Place a wide wooden board from the chair seat to the bed, so enabling the patient to slide into his chair. A suitable sliding board should be obtained from the hospital physical medicine department. The same methods, but in reverse, are used for getting the patient back into bed. It will again be seen that to perform these activities safely the patient needs to have good mobility and strong upper limbs.

*Can you tell me what kind of exercises I should do?*

It is of vital importance that the patient should continue to exercise at home. Instructions regarding this can be obtained from the physical medicine department of the patient's hospital.

*Can you help me to walk with my crutches?*

Yes, if you have had any experience at this; if not, it would be unwise to attempt it. Should the patient fall and damage his stump a long delay might result in his rehabilitation.

*Do you think I should have an artificial limb as I am so old?*

Many old patients do very well on artificial limbs, but this question can only be answered by the patient's medical officer. The home visitor should not become involved in this matter; it should be left to the doctor to decide.

The following list of questions and answers are those likely to be asked by the amputee who has received his temporary pylon or permanent limb. Many of the previous questions will also apply to this group.

*Now that I have my artificial leg can you teach me to walk on it at home?*

No, this must be done by a qualified therapist.

*Can you help me put my limb on?*

Yes, then follow the instructions given for the particular level of amputation. You must read the instructions carefully, as a badly applied limb will cause stump damage.

*My limb hurts me. Can you help?*

No, but advise the patient to make an appointment to attend his limb-fitting centre.

*My limb is in need of some repair. What should I do?*

Make an appointment to attend the limb-fitting centre. Do not attempt to make any adjustment to the limb; this must be done at the limb centre.

*Must I always wear this woollen sock over my stump?*
Yes, unless instructions have been given not to do so.

*I have lost my stump socks. Can I wear the limb without them?*
No, the patient must write to the limb-fitting centre for a further supply.

*Can you take me out in my wheelchair?*
Yes, if the patient has been told not to wear his limb, otherwise the patient should be encouraged to try walking short distances on his limb.

*My sticks are too short. Can you give me longer ones?*
No, the patient should report to his limb-fitting centre. It is not uncommon to find patients who believe that longer sticks will hold their backs up. This of course is untrue; it is the work of the extensor muscles of the spine.

*Now that I am wearing my limb all day how often should I bandage my stump?*
Follow the instructions given on stump bandaging.

*Now that I have my limb do I still apply to my hospital for another bandage?*
No, apply to the limb centre.

*My stump is very painful, should I go to the limb centre?*
No, the patient must first report to his medical officer.

*Can you show me how to climb the stairs and how to get up off the floor?*
No, the patient must be given these instructions by a qualified therapist. These are two strenuous activities and some patients, due to their physical health, are advised not to attempt such activities.

Many other problems may arise from home visits, but the home visitor is advised never to do anything by chance. When in doubt always consult the patient's medical officer.

# 7

# Corrective Exercise Therapy for Flexion Contractures of Hip and Knee Joints

Before going into details concerning exercise therapy for flexion contractures of the hip and knee joints, it would be well to explain some of the difficulties and time-consuming problems that these deformities present, thereby delaying early rehabilitation.

### FROM THE PROSTHETIC POINT OF VIEW

Some adjustment to the socket, or even a new socket, might have to be made. Considering that the degree of flexion contracture tends to increase from time to time, due to inactivity and lack of understanding, adjusting the socket could be an almost perpetual occurrence until further surgery was indicated or the patient became unsuited to an artificial limb.

With through-knee (disarticulation) stumps it is possible to move the weight load off the ischial tuberosity on to the natural weight-bearing surface of the femur, which makes good use of the proprioceptive impulses at the distal end of the stump. But these advantages are lost if a hip flexion contracture is present.

Contractures of the hip and knee joint may well confine the choice of limb to only one type.

### FROM THE PATIENT'S POINT OF VIEW

There may be some resentment over the appearance of the prosthesis which is not always aesthetically satisfying, especially to women. Sometimes a man is unable to get his trouser leg over the bulging socket. Amputees with long femoral stumps and hip flexion contractures find it difficult to sit up to a table with their limbs on. It must also be realized that it is much more difficult for an elderly person to walk safely on his prosthesis, or even to produce anything like an acceptable gait, if there is flexion deformity at the hip or knee joint. It is, therefore, vitally important that the therapist should take every precaution to prevent these deformities from occurring. Early exercise to the extensor and adductor groups of muscles working on the hip joint for the above-knee amputee, and to the extensors of knee and abductors of the hip for the below-knee amputees should be given. Correct bed and chair postures should also be taught with a simple explanation of why these are considered important.

However, the therapist may be required to treat amputees who have already developed contractures of the hip and knee joints, and a great deal of time can be wasted in attempts to correct them if the therapist is unaware of their history.

Flexion contractures of the hip and knee joints are classified as follows:

1. Non-remediable or permanent
2. Remediable or not permanent

### NON-REMEDIABLE CONTRACTURES

These are due to: (1) a bony block in the joint from injury, arthritis etc.; (2) soft tissue contractures due to scarring; (3) permanent contractures in the joint capsule, ligaments and muscles due to previous disease; (4) long periods of bad postural habits; (5) inadequate treatment during the remedial phase.

### REMEDIABLE CONTRACTURES

These are due to: (1) muscular imbalance caused by the division of muscles normally operating round the joint; (2) failure to maintain a correct postural position either before or after amputation.

### BASIC APPROACH

Before attempting any form of corrective exercise with patients with flexion contracture, it is important to ascertain whether the condition is remediable or not. The therapist who tries to correct the latter by exercise will only be wasting valuable time. The permanent contracture must be accepted as such, and the degree of flexion deformity accommodated in the socket of the limb. Certainly this is not ideal, but unfortunately experience has shown that in these cases surgery must be used as no amount of exercise alone will improve the deformity. It is suggested that for amputees in this category, periods of exercise to improve the exercise tolerance of the body generally and an early appointment at the patient's nearest limb-fitting centre are the best treatment.

Many other contractures, however, can be improved and every attempt should be made to do so. It is possible to reduce the degree of flexion deformity by exercise therapy and in some cases to restore full range of joint movement. Any amputee with a contracture of more than five degrees is at a disadvantage before he starts his prosthetic training. This is even more so in cases of below-knee amputees should there be contracture in both hip and knee joints.

It can be expected that those therapists involved in amputee rehabilitation will no doubt be faced both with patients who are attending for general exercise therapy and stump exercises prior to limb fitting and with those attending with a prosthesis for prosthetic training. In both instances contractures of the hip and knee joints may well be found.

Patients who have remediable contractures should be given a specific period of corrective exercise therapy and not simply be included in a 'stump class'. Obviously, these patients will take a little longer than others to become independent but if, finally, they are able to manage their prostheses better and more safely, if posture and gait are improved, the result will indeed be satisfying to both patient and therapist.

TECHNIQUES

The most common method of treating flexion contractures is that of passive stretching of the contracted muscle group by the therapist. It is, however, a painful and time-consuming method, and not very popular with the patient. If this method is to be used, the following points must be considered. Only by active shortening of the extensor muscles can we hope to reduce any flexion deformity. If the therapist is stretching the flexors passively, the patient should be attempting to extend his stump actively at the same time. But it is questionable whether the patient can in fact do this for his movement will be inhibited by pain caused by the stretching of the flexor muscles. It must be accepted that unless one group of muscles relaxes, or plays out, its antagonists cannot work. It is also unlikely that a patient could tolerate up to 30 minutes of passive stretching; anything less would be a waste of time. Other methods used are spring and weight resistance and periods with the patient lying prone on a low trolley. Each method has its quota of success but, unless each is given with care and physiological understanding, it will tend to delay early rehabilitation.

Flexion deformities are generally found in elderly patients, and some thought must be given to the possibility of their not being able to comprehend fully or to concentrate on their part of the exercise. Furthermore, their pain tolerance can be expected to be lower and they may quickly build up resentment towards what is to them a painful form of treatment. Elderly patients therefore make additional demands upon the skill and understanding of the therapist.

In the attempt to overcome possible difficulties of this sort all amputees with flexion contractures, and in particular the elderly, should first be given a specific period of relaxation to the lower extremities, with a clear and simple explanation of why it is necessary for the stump to be relaxed. This is followed by active extension exercises of the stump, starting from the fullest outer range. These should not be vigorous and the patient should be encouraged to extend a little further when the limit of extension has been reached. Progression is by attaching a spring or weight resistance to the extensor muscles, the resistance again starting from the outer range. This will gradually build up muscle power which, when followed by limb wearing, will ultimately eliminate a great deal, if not all, of the flexion contracture.

POSITION OF PATIENT

The most suitable position for the unilateral above-knee amputee is 'crook side lying', amputated side uppermost. The patient should be facing the wall-bars, or some other fitment, suitable later for the use of springs or weight resistance. A pillow is placed between the sound leg, or behind, to support the stump. This will encourage relaxation, prevent the stump from falling into adduction and provide a smooth surface for the stump to move over.

This position should be maintained until the patient is able to reach a true extension. From then on, the position should change to 'prone lying' for active extension exercises, thus using the resistance of gravity plus the weight of the stump. Stronger resisted exercises can then be introduced as a final means of progression in strength.

For the bilateral above-knee amputee the most practical position is lying 'supine'. This will, however, present two other problems that need observing. Firstly, care must be taken not to allow the weight of the stumps to cause any tension on the hip flexors and, secondly, any tendency to increase the lumbar curve must be avoided. To help avoid this it is suggested that the stumps might be suspended by overhead slings attached to light springs or be supported by rubber or sponge cushions. As a precaution against the possible increase of lumbar curve during the working phase, the patient should be encouraged to work each stump individually, holding one in full flexion while working the other. The position of the overhead springs must be fixed so that the resistance to the extensor muscles will start in the outer range.

Below-knee amputees with contracture of the knee joint can become a problem, particularly those with short stumps. They may well need some individual attention but too much time should not be wasted; provided that the hip joint has a full range of movement, the knee joint is of secondary importance. Where there is a good length of stump more time should be given to reducing the deformity, on the same principle as for the above-knee, building up the strength of the extensor muscles from within the outer range. However, priority must be given to the hip joint; there is little advantage in having two joints above the site of amputation if the hip joint has a limited range of movement.

The technique that has been discussed is a suitable form of corrective exercise therapy, specifically for contractures of the hip and knee joints; it offers the following advantages:

1. It is physiologically sound
2. It is active work by the patient with less pain
3. It is suitable for group work or the patient can work alone
4. The early phase could be carried out in the ward.

# 8

# Stump Bandaging

The importance of stump bandaging cannot be over-emphasized. Crêpe bandages are the most suitable.

5 m of 6 in bandage are required for above-knee stumps.

5 m of 4 in bandage are required for below-knee stumps. In cases where there is a long femoral stump it may be necessary to have two 6 in bandages sewn together, making a double length.

Many therapists will have had the opportunity of bandaging a stump in the early days following the removal of sutures and, no doubt, great care will have been taken not to cause the patient any unnecessary discomfort, knowing that the stump is still painful and that a tender scar is present. This caution, however, can easily be overdone and may well retard the patient's progress if correct stump bandaging is not started early. Where the cause of amputation has been vascular disease, when the stump takes longer to heal, tight bandaging should be delayed. It is not true to assume that the need for stump bandaging is to shape the stump. This is done by the surgeon performing the operation, and no amount of bandaging will alter the shape. The aims of stump bandaging are as follows:

1. To help reduce any terminal oedema
2. To encourage a healthy venous return
3. To help tone up flabby tissue
4. To avoid an adductor roll in the groin
5. To accustom the stump to a constant covering

These five aims are known as conditioning the stump for limb wearing.

## OEDEMA

Following amputation, most stumps show some terminal oedema which is due partly to the trauma of surgery, but the effect is magnified by the inevitable large dead space which communicates with cut muscle and bone and the divided lymphatic channels and by the gravitational position of the stump.

Unless assisted by some form of compression or support, this terminal oedema will disperse only slowly. In fact, stumps that have not been treated for this have been found, many months later, to show the indurated type of oedema; this delays the establishment of collateral circulation and may result in breakdown and ulceration.

Correct stump bandaging from the earliest possible time is the only means of assistance that can be applied to the stump for this purpose.

## ABOVE-KNEE STUMPS

The ideal position for the patient is that of lying supine on a couch or plinth. Using about 5 m of 6 in crêpe bandage, begin at the anterior aspect at the level of the inguinal ligament, the patient fixing each corner with his thumbs (Fig. 6). Proceed to cover, lengthwise, the stump and the lower extremity *centrally*; continue up the posterior aspect as far as the gluteal fold and have the patient fix the bandage with his fingers. Return to the starting position, this time covering the *lateral* aspect of the stump's extremity; fix again by patient's thumbs, and return once more to the gluteal fold, covering the *medial* aspect of the stump's extremity (Fig. 7).

These three layers should be firm but not tight. Now bandage from the *outside in* (this is most important), making the first diagonal turn from the *top outside* to the *bottom inside* of the stump (Fig. 8). Continue round the bottom of the stump to start a second diagonal turn from the *bottom outside* to the *top inside* of the stump (Fig. 9), making sure that the bandage is taken well into the groin. Continue to make two straight turns at the proximal end of the stump finishing with the bandage on the outside of the stump as in Fig. 10. Now repeat the first two diagonal turns, then pass the bandage under the buttock from the inside to the position shown in Fig. 11. Holding the bandage on the crest, continue over the abdomen and behind to cross on the

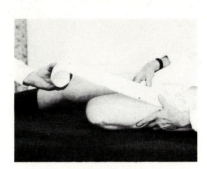

Fig. 6.

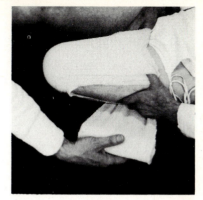

Fig. 7.

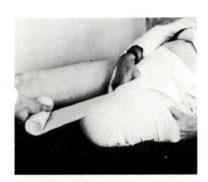

Fig. 8.

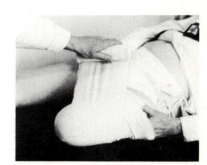

Fig. 9.

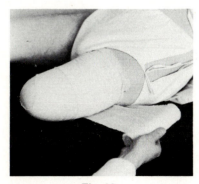

Fig. 10.

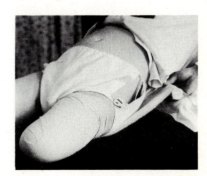

Fig. 11.

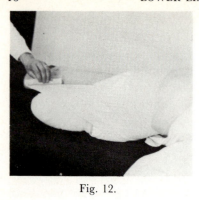

Fig. 12.

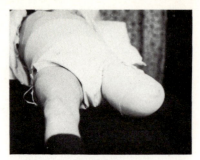

Fig. 13.

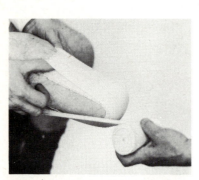

Fig. 14.

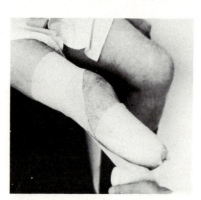

Fig. 15.

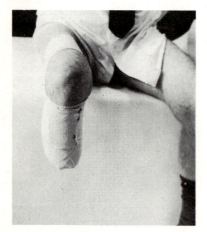

Fig. 16.

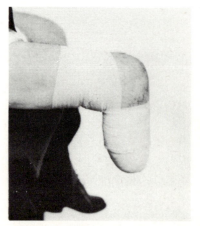

Fig. 17.

crest as in Fig. 12. Take the bandage down the inside of the stump and finish off by pinning the bandage in a suitable position (Fig. 13).

It is not possible to say just how much pressure should be applied—it depends entirely on the sensitivity of the stump. Only by constant repetition of stump bandaging can the therapist become able to assess the correct tension. It should be understood that unless the pressure is mainly at the distal end of the stump, decreasing slightly as the bandage reaches the groin, the desired end result will be delayed.

The bandage should be reapplied three times a day; morning, midday and at night. It should be worn during sleep and taken off during exercise.

This procedure is continued until the patient receives his prosthesis. While the prosthesis is being worn all day the bandaging may be discontinued, but if it is found that the patient is unable to get the limb on comfortably in the morning he should be instructed to put the bandage on again each night before going to bed. If, for any reason, the patient is taken off the limb for any length of time, then stump bandaging, morning and night, must be restarted.

## BELOW-KNEE STUMPS

The sitting position is the ideal one for the patient. Using 5 m of 4 in crêpe bandage, start at the anterior aspect at the level of the tibial tubercle, fixing the bandage with the patient's thumbs, and proceed as with the above-knee amputee, covering the central, lateral and medial aspects of the stump's extremity, the patient fixing the bandage posteriorly with his fingers at the level of the head of fibula (Fig. 14). Secure the bandage by taking two turns around the thigh just above the knee (Fig. 15) before pinning off (Figs 16, 17).

### SYME'S AMPUTATIONS

Bandaging the Syme's amputated stump is as for the below-knee stump, taking care not to displace the heel pad at the distal end of the stump.

## DISARTICULATION OF HIP AND HINDQUARTER AMPUTATIONS

The ideal position is for the patient to be standing or, failing this, crook side lying may be used, the amputated side being uppermost.

Using a 6 in bandage, begin by taking two turns around the waist, starting on the amputated side. Passing forward over the abdomen and behind, proceed to cover firmly the amputated area, using the waist to anchor the bandage.

In cases of disarticulation or a trans-trochenteric amputation, where there is pendulous tissue below the level of symphysis pubis, it is important that the bandage should be taken into the groin and that this pendulous tissue should not be allowed to adopt an abducted position.

### SOME IMPORTANT POINTS

1. For very smooth skin, a *crêpe* bandage is more serviceable.
2. When using an elastic bandage, use only at *half-stretch*.
3. When reapplying a bandage to the stump, first roll it up on the stretch and *use it in reverse*, starting with the end that was pinned.
4. Never attempt to use any bandage that has *lost its elasticity*. This is a waste of time.
5. For very short above-knee stumps, take two turns around the waist. Do *not* cut the bandage.
6. For very short below-knee stumps it is advisable to bandage the stump *in extension*, covering the whole of the knee.
7. Before bandaging any stump, examine the surrounding areas very carefully for any abrasions, *particularly in the groin*, and for any skin disorder.
8. Correct bandaging can solve many problems.
9. When bandaging a disarticulation of knee joint, or a Gritti–Stokes amputation, it is necessary to take the bandage up to the groin. If this is not done, some delay in limb fitting will follow.
10. For some above-knee stumps, particularly those short and fat, the above technique is not always satisfactory. Other methods

should, therefore, be used provided that (a) the stump is not pulled into flexion, (b) the bandage has been taken up into the groin, (c) it has been applied firmly and (d) it will stay on overnight.

# Part Two

# The Prosthetic and Late Phase of Treatment

# 9

# First Visit to the Limb Centre

The first visit to the limb-fitting centre is made after a request form or letter has been sent to the centre by the hospital or by the patient's own doctor. A limb-fitting file is then opened and an appointment made for the patient to attend for examination.

On arrival, the patient is allocated to one of the limb medical officers. A routine examination of the stump is made in order to ascertain its condition and a history of the patient is taken. With the required information at his disposal, the medical officer can decide which type of prosthesis will be best suited to the patient. An order prescription form is completed either for a temporary (pylon) prosthesis or for a permanent articulated limb.

The patient is then given an opportunity of choosing which limb maker he wishes for his artificial limb. If he is in doubt he can visit a showroom and see sample limbs of the type he needs which have been made by several limb makers under contract to the Government. Having made his choice, he is taken to the fitting room to begin the late stage of rehabilitation.

It is as well to mention here that not all patients get as far as this on their first visit; some are sent back to the hospital with a request for further stump bandaging and physical treatment.

BASIC PROCEDURE OF FIRST VISIT TO THE LIMB MAKERS

The patient arrives with the order prescription form from the limb medical officer. The prescription contains a specification either for a temporary pylon or for a fully articulated permanent prosthesis. He is then received by the prosthetist who proceeds to take measurements and profiles of both the amputated side and the sound side;

in addition, for certain sites of amputation, a plaster cast is taken of the stump.

Casting technique calls for applied pressures and markings on anatomical lines for the various types of prosthesis prescribed. Measurements are taken for checking and cross-checking, the sound limb measurements being taken for cosmetic reasons and for duplication on the prosthesis. The patient is asked to supply a shoe into which the artificial foot is fitted (but not in the case where a pylon is indicated). Using these specifications the prosthesis is made in the workshop ready for the fitting stage (second visit); the limb is fitted to the patient by the prosthetist, and then returned to the workshop for completion and delivery. On his third visit the patient with the limb on is referred back to the ordering limb medical officer for checking and passing out as satisfactory.

Each prosthetist is a highly skilled man and undergoes a long period of training before being authorized to take casts and measurements and to fit the many sites of amputations which range from hindquarter, disarticulations, above- and below-knees, Syme's and Chopart's foot amputations, and many congenital deformities.

It cannot be left unsaid that the prosthetist, although employed by a private contractor, is a vital member of the rehabilitation team. Therapists should not hesitate to meet and discuss their problems with the prosthetist.

# 10

# First Principles of Prosthetic Training Techniques

It will be appreciated that there are many types of artificial limb. It has been decided, therefore, to include a chapter on each common site of amputation, discussing the techniques used and some of the problems that face the amputee. Unfortunately, it is not possible to discuss every problem that arises, and *it will be appreciated that every amputee is an individual and must be treated as such*. The information given, therefore, must be adapted to individual requirements.

Basically, there is a set pattern that should be followed, from the patient's first attendance to the end of his treatment, when he becomes once again a normal member of the community. This latter requirement must be the primary aim, whether the patient is to return to work or just remain independent and safe.

The first thing that comes to mind is the responsibility that eventually passes to the therapist who has to educate the amputee in the use of his prosthesis. He is the last member of a team of professional people who have played a part in the total rehabilitation, and it is this therapist who is ultimately expected to obtain a good result.

The surgeon cannot always oblige by making the site of amputation an ideal one from the prosthetic point of view, so that the prosthetist is often faced with either a very short stump or, as in the cases of hindquarter and disarticulation of the hip joint, no stump at all. When these problems arise, conditions for early rehabilitation are not ideal, but they cannot be avoided and must be dealt with in the best possible way.

It must not be assumed that patients who fall into one of the two previously mentioned categories will not do well. Most disarticulations and hindquarter amputations do very well indeed, it is often just a matter of time. For those with very short stumps automatic knee locks can be fitted, giving early stability and security. With correct exercises in balancing and prosthetic training, they soon learn to manage the prosthesis effectively.

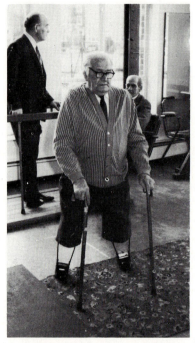

Fig. 18. A small section of the amputee unit at Clayton Hospital showing a unilateral above-knee amputee in the walking rails and a bilateral above-knee amputee on rocker pegs taking his first steps over a carpet.

## CHILDREN AND THEIR PROSTHESES

Most children take readily to limb wearing and very quickly learn to get from one place to another. The gait may not be graceful, particularly if the knee joint is absent, but independence is quickly achieved and the prosthesis accepted. This acceptance is most important.

No minimum age has been recognized for beginning limb fitting, the first limb generally being supplied when the child begins to stand on the sound limb (or on the stumps, in bilateral amputees); this usually happens at ten to twelve months.

For infants no walking training is given following delivery of the limb. Parents are instructed in the application of the limb and encouraged to keep the prosthesis with the child's toys etc., putting it on to the stump as often as possible. In this way the child soon becomes accustomed to handling and recognizing its purpose.

When the child is a little older and responsive to instruction, a course of prosthetic training can be given to iron out any bad faults or habits.

Almost every child is at first supplied with an all-wood limb. This is lighter in weight than metal, and easier to lengthen simply by dividing and keying in a further piece of the required length. The wooden shin piece will survive a great deal of rough treatment with little effect on its efficiency. The ankle joint is fixed at this stage and ensures stability, up to the age of about eight years. There is, however, some movement in the toe joint area. A felt foot is most commonly used.

## APPENDAGES

In view of the fact that the pelvis is not fully developed, pelvic bands and waist belts are generally omitted and a three-point shoulder suspension is provided.

Progress to the standard type of prosthesis is decided by the limb medical officer. It may be at adolescence or earlier. A further course of prosthetic training is then given if necessary but, whatever the site of amputation, the technique of training will be the same as that already given.

# 11

# Prosthetic Training Techniques

## UNILATERAL ABOVE-KNEE

It is impossible for any patient to walk well if the prosthesis is not a good fit. It is advisable, therefore, to check the application to see that it has been made correctly, as a badly applied limb will only result in a long delay. With some patients it is necessary to check the application at every attendance as attempts are often made to pack the socket; bandages, cotton-wool and underclothes are sometimes used for this purpose. This procedure causes the stump to ride very high and results in pain, difficulty in lifting the limb off the ground, circumduction and internal rotation.

When applying the prosthesis the stump is covered by one woollen sock only, which is pulled well up into the groin and then placed well into the socket, with the limb in slight external rotation. The pelvic band is buckled together firmly in the front, passing round and above the iliac crest of the opposite side. The fastening of the pelvic band should correct the alignment of the foot to the forward position.

The shoulder strap is placed over the opposite shoulder and clipped on to the pelvic band, front and back; this should not be tight. The stump sock is pulled up and turned over the lip of the socket all round. It should not be allowed to slip back into the socket; if this does occur a longer sock should be used.

It is most important to make sure that patients attending for prosthetic training on a pylon for the first time are wearing a normal outdoor shoe on the sound limb and not a house slipper. This is often found to be the cause of their complaining that the pylon is too long.

All patients should be measured for their prostheses while standing in a normal shoe, the height of the heel being taken into account. The patient who arrives for training wearing a slipper should be asked if he was wearing the slipper when measured. If not, a normal shoe should be obtained before training begins. Sometimes the patient arrives at the limb centre for measuring direct from the hospital ward, wearing only pyjamas, dressing-gown and a slipper. The prosthetist will measure him, allowing for the height of a heel, and will explain to the patient that he must wear a normal shoe on his next visit. Unfortunately, this sound advice is seldom followed.

Circumstances do arise, however, where it is found that the patient has been measured to the height of the slipper, and so when he wears a normal shoe the limb appears short due to the extra height of the heel. This should not cause immediate alarm as the limb can be quickly lengthened. Far fewer bad gaits arise from limbs that are too short than from those that are too long.

## TESTING FOR A GOOD FIT

The patient stands wearing the limb and the therapist places a finger on the ischial tuberosity and asks the patient to ease his weight off the limb. Next, the limb is brought into extension behind him; he is then told to let the limb bear his full weight. The ischial tuberosity should rest directly over the ischial seating provided on the limb. If it is found that the tuberosity has passed inside the socket and causes pain on the adductor tendon, it may be assumed that stump shrinkage has taken place and an extra stump sock will be required. If the patient has to wear three socks for comfort, the socket should be relined by the prosthetist, and *one* sock only should then be worn. If, on the other hand, it is found that the tuberosity is more than 2.5 cm (1 in) above the tuber seating, it may be assumed that the stump size has increased. There are two solutions to this problem: (1) additional stump bandaging and exercises, (2) a thin cotton sock may be worn and pulled down from the inside while the patient is weight-bearing. This may pull the surplus tissues into the socket sufficiently to enable normal prosthetic training to be followed. Failing this, the limb medical officer may order an adjustment to be made to the socket.

At the beginning, whether the fitting be good or bad, the majority of patients usually complain of a burning sensation in the area of the ischial tuberosity. This will subside within one or two weeks provided the limb is worn every day. However, while this discomfort persists the patient will have difficulty in walking. With emaciated patients it may be necessary to have a sorbo-rubber pad covering the ischial seating to encourage full weight-bearing.

A further sorbo-rubber pad known as a touch-bearing pad may be found fitted into the bottom of the socket, particularly in the primary above-knee pylon. Its purpose is to encourage a more efficient circulatory flow at the distal end of the stump by the piston action which occurs during walking. The stump presses slightly on to the pad during weight-bearing and is released when non-weight-bearing. This creates a pumping or massage effect on the tissues, resulting in a warm and less tender stump.

### PELVIC SUSPENSION

The normal pelvic suspension found on the above-knee pylon or permanent prosthesis is known as a 'ridged pelvic band' (Fig. 19), its primary aim being to stabilize the limb on the patient. The limb will remain safe and secure with the minimum amount of muscle work, permitting the fullest possible range of flexion and extension of the hip joint, a limited range of abduction and adduction. Rotation can be achieved only by rotating the complete pelvis on the hip joint of the sound side, with the prosthesis off the ground. Any rotation with the limb weight-bearing becomes a pivot, and this should not be permitted.

### DOUBLE SWIVEL PELVIC BAND

This type of suspension seen in Fig. 20 will be found only on the permanent articulated prosthesis, and is supplied at the discretion of the limb medical officer to those patients presenting the ideal above-knee stump—*good length, full range of hip movement* and *muscular*. These requirements would indicate that the stump would be capable of controlling and stabilizing the limb to a sound margin of safety. The double swivel pelvic band will permit a complete full range of hip movements to be carried out on the prosthesis.

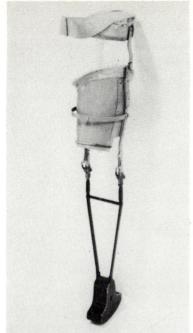

Fig. 19. Above-knee temporary pylon with ridged pelvic band.

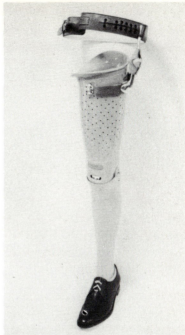

Fig. 20. Above-knee permanent prosthesis with double swivel pelvic band.

### WEBBING WAIST BELT AND THREE-POINT SUSPENSION

This type of suspension is generally found on the temporary below-knee pylon (Fig. 21) and the temporary through-knee pylon. In Figs 30 and 31 it will be seen that the permanent prostheses for these two levels of amputation are supplied without any form of lateral stability as there would be if a rigid pelvic band had been fitted. Therefore, the training on the pylon suspended by the waist belt and three-point suspension will help the limb medical officer to decide whether or not the patient will manage a permanent limb of the P.T.B. type for the below-knee amputee, or a permanent through-knee limb with a leather corset. Therapists will now see why it is so important that the abductor muscles of the amputated side are exercised strongly to stabilize the hip joint when taking weight on the prosthesis.

Above-knee amputees may well have this type of suspension for their pylon, and provided that they have good muscular control over the pylon it will enhance their ability on their permanent prosthesis.

Problems arising from the pelvic suspensions are few; generally they concern the application. The ridged pelvic band which opposes the iliac crest will cause some discomfort if the underclothes are not smoothed out, or if the pelvic band is too loose, so permitting friction

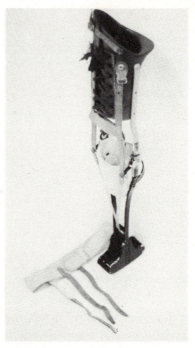

Fig. 21.    Below-knee temporary pylon with adjustable leather corset, waistbelt and three-point suspension.

between the joint and the iliac crest. In some instances it may be thought that the pelvic band is too low, but a closer examination will show that the patient has padded himself well out of the socket trying to ease the pressure off his ischial tuberosity.

The double swivel pelvic band may offer a similar problem as above, but this is rare. One difficulty may well be revealed in the early days; the patient complains that he feels the limb fall away from him as he starts to swing the leg forward. Examination will show that the patient's stump has reduced in size and is now too loose in the socket, or that, due to the bucket handle type of attachment of the pelvic band to the socket, the patient may experience a slight drop of the limb as he begins to swing it forward. This will improve as the muscles become accustomed to controlling the limb.

With the waist belt and three-point suspension, most patients complain that they cannot prevent the limb from rotating inwardly. There are several causes of this. First check that the limb has been put on correctly, turned slightly outward and the corset laced firmly. The suspension straps must fall in line with the buckles and be fixed firmly. Second, check that the patient is not rotating his hip joint inwardly as he takes a step with his pylon. Finally, the stump may have increased in size and no longer be fitting the socket.

## THE SUCTION SOCKET LIMB

Suction socket limbs can be issued at the discretion of the limb medical officer to patients with above-knee stumps which are of suitable length with well toned-up muscles and with no circulatory problems.

The socket may be of either metal or wood. The shape and fitting of the suction socket differ somewhat from the normal above-knee socket inasmuch as it is shaped to the muscle contour of the stump. As the muscles contract, the limb remains firmly attached to the stump. A two-way suction valve is situated on the lower lateral aspect of the socket.

When weight-bearing takes place, air is pushed out through the valve. As the weight is taken off, a certain amount of air is admitted so as to avoid a complete vacuum.

Application of this limb is best done standing. A long thin cotton sock is first pulled over the stump. The free end of the sock is placed inside the socket and pushed through the hole on the lower lateral aspect. The stump is now placed into the socket, and while weight-bearing the cotton sock is pulled off the stump through the bottom hole. The valve is screwed into place and the leg is then firmly fixed. Prosthetic training for the suction socket wearer is the same as that for single above-knee amputees. During the first few days of limb wearing, a regular check of the stump's extremity to observe if there is any circulatory disturbance is always helpful.

## BASIC PRINCIPLES OF PROSTHETIC TRAINING (WITH PYLON)

*First Attendance.* The whole of this period is spent in the walking rails perfecting the following exercises:

1. Standing balance, pylon slightly backwards
2. Hip updrawing of amputated side (Fig. 22)
3. Transferring of weight from one leg to the other, first in the *stride standing* position, then in the *walk forward* position. Alternating the position of the pylon, forward and backward (Fig. 23)

The body should always be erect; if it is not erect, the shoulder strap should be checked for tightness and the hip checked for flexion contracture.

*Second Attendance.* Exercises as above, introducing three-point walking, i.e. both hands forward, followed by prosthesis, then the sound leg.

*Third Attendance.* Three-point walking, with correction of posture, gait, even paces and full weight-bearing.

*Fourth Attendance.* Four-point walking in the rails, i.e. right hand forward, left leg forward, left hand forward, right leg forward.

*Fifth Attendance.* Four-point walking with stick in one hand, other hand on rail. The stick should change hands alternately.

*Finally.* Four-point walking with two sticks, progressing out of the rails to practising the following functional activities: free walking; sitting down and getting up from chair; stair-climbing; walking up and down inclines; falling and getting up off mattress; stepping over and around obstacles; walking backwards and sideways; walking in a crowd and picking up small articles from the floor.

At all times patients must be encouraged to brace the stump back into extension when weight-bearing. As previously explained, the sequence of instruction should be modified to individual requirements.

## STICKS

Two sticks or none? This is a topic in which the therapist invariably finds himself involved, and the suggested solution is this: it must be realized that there is a fundamental difference between a patient recovering from a fractured femur, for instance, and one who has

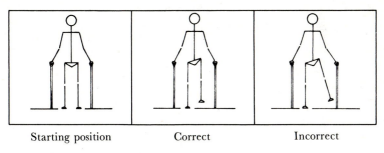

Starting position      Correct      Incorrect

Fig. 22. Hip updrawing.

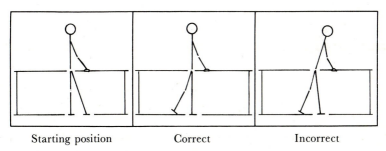

Starting position      Correct      Incorrect

Fig. 23. Transferring body weight (walk forward position). Pylon in front.

lost a limb, whether it be above or below the knee. The absence of a limb takes a great deal of getting used to; therefore the amputee should be encouraged to use only one stick which should be held in the opposite hand.

Most patients soon learn that they can help themselves more readily with one free hand, but it takes time at this early stage on the pylon. By the time the patient has received his articulated limb he will be more easily weaned away from his sticks, having had more time to get used to his pylon.

It would be unfair for anyone to suggest that any individual patient should throw away his sticks at a specified time. This is a psychological problem for the patient, not a mechanical one. Good balance, correct training and encouragement are needed, and the sticks will soon disappear.

### LENGTH OF STICKS

An incorrect length of stick can easily retard a patient's progress, apart from causing possible postural defects. The correct stick length is found by first having the patient standing upright with arms hanging loosely by his side. The stick is then placed vertically by his side, ferrule uppermost. A mark is made on the stick at a level with the ulnar styloid process. The stick is then shortened to this point and the ferrule reattached.

This procedure should provide the patient with a stick of the correct length for weight-bearing.

### UNILATERAL, ABOVE-KNEE WITH ARTICULATED LIMB

More often than not it will be found that most of the older patients, and those with a weak stump in particular, are supplied with a prosthesis which has a semi-automatic knee lock. This locks as the patient stands up and extends the stump, and is easily released when he requires to flex the knee in order to sit down. With this type of limb the technique of training is the same as for the pylon.

### ARTICULATED KNEE JOINT

On the first day the patient is taken to the walking rails. He should be instructed not to interfere with the wheel-type control mechanism which can be found on the side or the anterior aspect of the knee. This control has been set by the prosthetist at the correct friction level, and should it become loose the patient may easily fall. On the other hand, should it become too tight the lower anterior aspect of the stump may become bruised and tender. It should also be made quite clear to the patient that this knee control unit should not be used as a device for permanently locking the knee joint.

With this type of limb we now have to break down the habit of hip updrawing and the patient is taught the following.

1. *Knee Flexion Control.* Standing between the rails , alternate knee flexion, keeping the feet on the ground, being certain that the heel of the artificial limb is firmly on the ground with full weght-bearing before flexing the sound knee (Fig. 24). (Adjustment of the elastic pick-up on the front of the limb, if necessary, will help to perfect this exercise.)

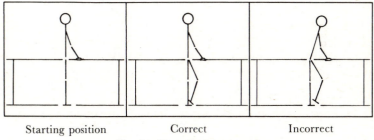

Starting position        Correct        Incorrect

Fig. 24. Knee flexion control.

2. *Single Step-taking.* (a) The artificial limb is placed behind the sound leg with full weight-bearing; (b) the body weight is then transferred on to the sound leg, the toe of the artificial limb remaining on the ground; (c) the artificial limb is *kicked* forward, the heel being placed on the ground just in front of the sound leg; (d) the stump is braced into the back of the socket, the knee kept fully extended; the artificial limb is returned to the starting position and the procedure is repeated (Fig. 25).

Having mastered these two exercises, continuity of walking may be started. It is now possible to observe any tendency for the patient to circumduct his limb by the alignment of the knee as it passes forward and beneath the body (Fig. 26). If there is a slight circumduction, check (a) the fitting, (b) the length and (c) abduction contracture of hip.

These are the three main causes of a circumducted gait which is a habit difficult to eliminate.

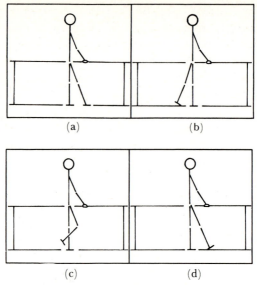

Fig. 25. Single step-taking.
(a) Starting position—artificial limb backward
(b) Phase 1—transferring body weight
(c) Phase 2—the swing-through
(d) Phase 3—placing heel down and forward

GAIT AND POSTURE

Without question it is the therapist's responsibility to try to obtain the best possible gait and posture from every patient. This, however, is easier said than done when dealing with elderly amputees, many

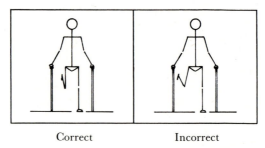

Correct            Incorrect

Fig. 26.   The swing-through seen from front view.

of whom have already developed a poor pattern of walking before their amputation, for reasons other than just getting old.

The therapist will find that a great deal of time is needed for trying to break down these bad habits of walking, plus teaching how to manage a prosthesis. It is suggested that provided that these patients are independent and safe on their limbs the question of gait and posture is only of secondary importance. Furthermore, to continue calling them into the amputee unit for treatment merely to try to improve their gait and posture will tend only to delay the programme of early rehabilitation.

For the younger and fit amputees the many problems of gait and posture seldom arise. The prosthetist is presented with good material to which to fit a prosthesis and is able to achieve a 100 per cent alignment on the limb, thus making it possible for these patients to obtain a good walking pattern in the shortest possible time during prosthetic training.

Most therapists take great pride in their efforts to reach a high standard of rehabilitation with each amputee. However, this enthusiasm should be tempered to the needs of each patient, bearing in mind that their first wish is to be able to help themselves at home with independence and safety. For some, such as the elderly, this may well be their only purpose, and more ambitious training could easily cause them anxiety and distress.

### FOOT RUBBERS

Occasionally a patient will complain of the limb being too long. He will say that he is unable to put his full weight on it while walking and yet finds it is comfortable when standing. It will be observed that while such patients are walking either they are not getting full extension of the hip or else the knee is continuously flexing slightly (knee shoot). This may well be due to the fact that the foot rubbers are too hard and so prevent the ankle joint from moving freely. If this is so, it is a job for the prosthetist, but it should first be reported to the limb medical officer for his permission to have the adjustment made.

### BLATCHFORD STABILIZED KNEE JOINT (B.S.K.)

The B.S.K. is now an alternative component to the standard central knee control unit found in almost every standard above-knee articulated prosthesis. It is supplied at the discretion of the limb medical officer.

It is not necessary here to explain the mechanism of this knee unit for the technique of prosthetic training is the same. The therapist should however be aware of its function and the advantages it can offer to the patient. It eliminates the need for additional knee-locking devices, because when full weight-bearing is taken on the limb with the knee joint in extension the joint is fully stable. Alternatively, with the knee joint flexed at any angle between approximately 5° to 35° with the full body weight over the knee joint centre, the flexed knee will support the body. To extend or to continue flexing the knee joint further, the weight must be taken off the limb. During the action of walking, bracing of the stump back into the socket need not be so vigorous, and consequently the managing of the prosthesis becomes less tiring. With the correct understanding of this knee unit such activities as climbing stairs or inclines, sitting and standing from a chair are made easier and safer.

It is not advisable to try to explain this type of mechanism to the patient during the first few days of training; it will only lead to confusion and delay. The patient will quickly appreciate the benefits for himself. The therapist, having given the basic instructions of prosthetic training, need only ensure that the patient is not walking and weight-bearing on permanently flexed knee and on the ball of his foot.

# 12

# Functional Activities for Unilateral Above-knee Amputees

SITTING DOWN AND STANDING UP FROM A CHAIR

*Sitting.* This may seem to be a simple thing to do, but with some patients instructions are necessary. The patient is taught to approach the chair from an angle, his sound leg being nearest the chair. When reaching the chair the sound leg is placed forward with full weight-bearing on it. The hand of the same side is placed on the seat or arm of the chair. The sound knee is slowly flexed and the body is lowered on to the chair. If the artificial knee joint is locked it is advisable to permit the patient to sit down first, then unlock the knee, until such time as he has achieved a good single leg balance, when he may be encouraged to free the knee while standing by extending the limb, and weight-bearing on the toe of the artificial limb. Care must be taken to see that the hand is so placed on the chair that it will not tip over.

During the procedure of sitting down, some patients will complain of pinching between the pelvic band and the top of the socket. If this cannot be overcome by teaching the patient to sit down with a 'straight back', so preventing too much hip flexion or by using a higher chair, the matter should be reported to the prosthetist through the limb medical officer.

*Standing Up.* If the patient is unable to push up from a chair by the use of both hands and his sound leg, he should reverse the actions of sitting down, first extending the knee of the prosthesis, turning slightly to the sound side and placing the hand of the sound side on the seat or arm of the chair. The stick in the other hand is placed *in front* of the artificial leg. The patient should push up with sound leg and hand, bracing the stump into extension; this action should result in his standing in the stride position, with the stick forming a three-point triangular base.

Patients should be instructed not to push on the stick as this will only cause a resistance to the body being raised out of the chair.

STAIR-CLIMBING

For the average unilateral above-knee amputee it is 'up with the sound leg leading, down with the artificial leg leading', offering very little problem at all; but we often come across the not-so-good sound leg, e.g. arthrodesis of hip or knee, calipers etc. The answer is to experiment and the easiest method found should be used. It is very difficult these days to find accommodation without stairs to climb

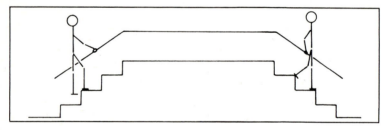

Fig. 27.     Unilateral above-knee amputee negotiating stairs. Note position of the feet.

and, therefore, very important that every patient should have the opportunity of trying every method before being told that he cannot manage stairs.

It is probably true to say that the above observations apply to all amputees except cases of cardiac failure, gross deformities, or other conditions where strenuous effort is contraindicated.

WALKING UP AND DOWN AN INCLINE

Any patient who finally gets out and about on his artificial limb must, at some time or other, be faced with walking up and down an incline. By simply crossing the road he may well find himself faced with this problem, and the very slightest camber of a road may cause the patient to fall.

To overcome this, the following method is suggested. Teach the patient to go up the incline, leading with the sound leg at each step and not allowing the prosthesis to come in front. Coming down should be the reverse, always leading with the prosthesis, and keeping the knee firmly braced in extension.

Many patients will manage quite well by putting one foot in front of the other, as in normal walking; these, it will be found, generally have good control of their stumps. If, at any time, the incline is found to be too steep for this method they should walk sideways, using the same sequence, with small steps.

## ESCALATORS

A great number of patients find it necessary to use escalators. This cannot be taught in the amputee unit, but they can be told that the safest method is to step on and off the escalator with the sound leg first.

## GETTING ON AND OFF PUBLIC TRANSPORT

Here again, for the good average unilateral amputee, there is no real problem at all. He will simply step up on to and down from the platform as in climbing stairs, sound leg up, artificial leg down. However, there are many who are deprived of travelling because, having succeeded in getting on to the bus, they find that the platform is too high for them when stepping down.

These patients should be taught to step down from a high platform backwards. Most public transport buses have two hand rails on the platform; using these as supports, patients can usually lower themselves on to their artificial leg. It is, of course, advisable for these patients to travel when possible during non-rush-hour periods.

## STEPPING OVER OBSTACLES

It cannot be considered a wise and practical procedure to encourage above-knee amputees, particularly elderly patients, to step *over* obstacles that are more than 15 cm high or wider than 10 cm, since a situation may arise in which the patient is in danger of being thrown off his balance due to the difficulty of having to swing the locked limb through a wide circumducted movement before being able to place his limb down on the other side of the obstacle.

With amputees using the free knee it may appear a little easier by the swing-through, but it must be remembered that the higher the thigh piece comes up, the less control can be kept over the foot; the shin piece will fall at right-angles to the thigh whether the patient steps over the obstacles with his sound leg first or his artificial leg.

It is, of course, necessary to include this functional activity in the programme of prosthetic training, but it is essential to keep the height of the obstacle only so high as to allow the patient's foot to pass over it after he has performed the movement of hip updrawing and hip flexing, as in taking a normal step forward. Those with a free knee will find this height manageable by the normal swing-through action.

To overcome the problem of negotiating high obstacles it is suggested that the patient should be taught to step on and off as in stair climbing, i.e. going up with the sound leg first and then down with the artificial limb first.

FALLING

It is true to say that the fear of falling lingers far longer in the mind of the patient than any other problem. This can be reduced to a great extent if he is influenced, by gentle persuasion and encouragement from the therapist, to fall on to a mattress several times before being discharged from the walking class. If one patient can be encouraged to demonstrate this act, it will be surprising to see how many others are willing to try, having seen one of their kind fall and get up unhurt.

A great deal of discretion must be used by the therapist when choosing his patient for this demonstration, e.g. any contraindications to strenuous effort will preclude a patient from acting as demonstrator.

Take the patient up to the mattress, instruct him to release his sticks quickly, fall on to his hands, and relax as he lets himself go. It will be noticed that most patients with a stiff knee prosthesis will fall and turn slightly to their sound side, flexing their sound knee. Those with a free knee will fall, flexing both knees, taking the prone kneeling position for a short time before rolling on to their sound side.

If these movements can be practised often, it will certainly help to reduce the possibility of serious injury following a genuine fall.

### GETTING UP FROM THE FLOOR

The patient takes up the long sitting position, gathering up his sticks and placing them on his sound side, the handles nearest his feet. He should then roll over on to his sound knee, the artificial limb extending backwards. By pushing up with his hands on to the sound leg, bringing the sticks up at the same time, he can then regain his balance and start walking (Fig. 28).

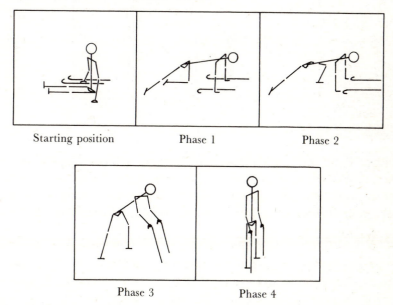

Starting position      Phase 1      Phase 2

Phase 3      Phase 4

Fig. 28. Unilateral above-knee amputee getting up from the floor.

### PICKING UP OBJECTS FROM THE FLOOR

For the average unilateral amputee this activity offers no problem. He extends the artificial leg backwards, flexes the sound knee and picks up the required object.

The following method can be taught to less confident unilateral amputees and also to bilateral amputees.

The patient adopts the stride standing position, approximately 0.7 m away from the required object. Both sticks are held forward

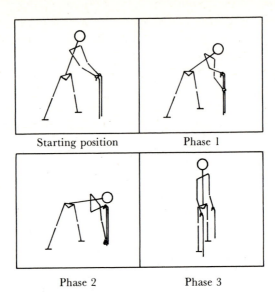

Starting position        Phase 1

Phase 2        Phase 3

Fig. 29.   Unilateral or bilateral amputee picking up small objects from the floor.

in one hand to form a three-point triangular base. The free hand
slides down the stick to maintain balance; while flexing the hips the
object is picked up and the patient returns in the same way to a
standing position. For bilateral amputees it is important that the
knee joints should be kept extended; if locks are fitted to the limbs,
they should be applied first.

It must be appreciated that this method can be used only for picking up small objects. In normal practice most bilateral amputees
prefer to wait until someone else comes along; nevertheless, it is
worth teaching, and the therapist can consider that he has fulfilled
his duty.

WALKING ON A CARPET

Many amputees, particularly those wearing a temporary pylon or
locked knee prosthesis, will complain that the limb sticks to the carpet causing them to fall. The reason for this is that either the action
of hip updrawing before placing the limb forward (hip flexion) has
not taken place or it has not been high enough for the base of the
foot or the rocker to move forward clear of the carpet pile. Con-

sequently, the patient feels that the limb is held fast by the carpet or sticking to the ground. Repetitive hip updrawing exercises with an explanation that the patient must transfer the body-weight on to the sound leg first will soon correct this problem.

# 13

# Below-knee Prostheses

There are several types of permanent below-knee limb, on which a brief description of their correct application is necessary.

1. Light metal below-knee limb, with leather thigh corset and sliding leather socket fitted into the container (shin piece) (Fig. 30).
2. Light metal below-knee limb, with blocked leather tuber-bearing thigh corset and sliding socket (Fig. 31).

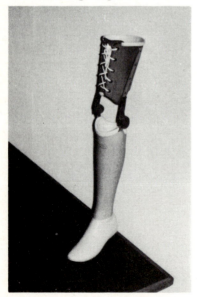

Fig. 30. Metal below-knee permanent limb with short corset.

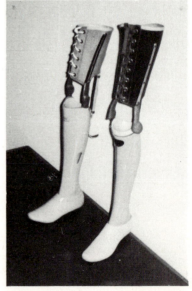

Fig. 31. Metal below-knee limb with tuber-bearing thigh corset (*right*). Wood below-knee pernament limb (*left*).

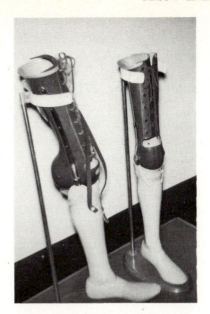

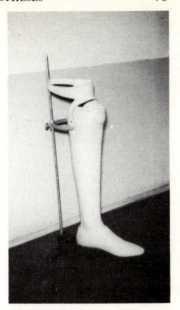

Fig. 32. Below-knee kneeling prosthesis (*right*). Through-knee end-bearing prosthesis (*left*).

Fig. 33. Below-knee patella tendon-bearing limb, with cuff
suspension.

3. All wood below-knee limb, with leather corset, with or without tuber seating, no sliding socket (Fig. 32).

4. Patella tendon-bearing below-knee limb, plastic or wood shin piece, with plastic socket, single cross-knee strap (cuff suspension) (Fig. 33).

APPENDAGES

For Types 1, 2 and 3 it is usual to find a web waist belt attached to the corset by elastic strap posteriorly and leather Y-shaped pick-up anteriorly.

In some instances these appendages may differ, but all will have the elastic strap and leather pick-up attachment. With the patella tendon-bearing below-knee limb there is the cross-knee strap (cuff suspension) or elastic stocking.

## APPLICATION OF PERMANENT PROSTHESIS

1. The weight-bearing area of this type of prosthesis is divided

between the condyles of the tibia and the thigh corset. There is no direct-weight bearing on the distal end of the stump. It will be appreciated that if the corset is assisting weight-bearing, it must be laced up firmly.

Cover the stump and the thigh with one woollen sock, place the stump through the corset into the socket and loosely lace the corset. Instruct the patient to stand up, pull up the sock and roll it over the edge of the corset all round. Place the knee in extension and instruct the patient to bear his full weight on the prosthesis.

The lower edge of the patella should be approximately 1 cm (0.5 in) above the anterior edge of the socket.

The patient then sits down, *maintaining the downward thrust of his stump into the socket*. Lace up the corset firmly; fix appendages. The leather pick-up should be sufficiently tight to assist the quadriceps in extending the knee.

It will easily be seen whether the stump has increased in size and therefore not fitting the socket, or whether shrinkage has taken place and the patella is either resting on or below the anterior edge of the socket.

Whatever the case, the remedy is the same as for the above-knee stumps: further bandaging and exercises, or adjustment of the socket.

2. The tuber-bearing seating on the corset of this limb would indicate that the stump is unfit for weight-bearing, or that there is some circulatory factor that contraindicates a tightly laced corset.

In appearance, the fitting of this limb is the same as the one described above, but full weight-bearing is taken on the ischial tuberosity.

Application of this limb is best done standing; first buckle up the strap at the top of the corset to keep the tuber seating in place; then, with the patient sitting, lace up the corset and fix appendages.

In view of the blocked leather corset and the fact that the stump is, so to speak, suspended in the socket, patients take a little longer to get used to their limb.

3. This type of prosthesis is very little different from those described above, with the exception that there is no separate socket and the stump fits directly into the shin piece.

Whether a patient is given a wood or metal limb is decided by the limb surgeon. The following factors, however, would indicate the possible issue of a wooden limb: stumps longer than 14 cm (5.5 in); hot climates and if the limb is intended for a child. Certain occupations also make a wooden limb preferable.

4. The patella tendon-bearing limb. Following a long series of experimental stages, the P.T.B. has been accepted by the Government as part of the National Health Service issue for below-knee amputees with suitable stumps, and has quickly taken over the role of becoming the standard below-knee limb in this country.

An outstanding feature of this limb is that the stump is held permanently in some slight degree of flexion within the socket. A close analysis of normal walking action will show that full extension of the knee joint takes place only for a brief moment, when full weight-bearing is taken through the joints; it is during this short period that full weight-bearing is taken on the patella tendon with no loss of stability to the amputee.

Likewise, in the normal standing position the knees are seldom fully extended unless the individual is standing to attention, which is not likely to happen to any amputee. The advantages of this limb are as follows: there is no leather thigh corset, so that bulk and weight are reduced. No resistance is offered to the thigh circulation, a circumstance which is very important in vascular conditions. No resistance is offered to further development of the quadriceps as when thigh corsets are laced too tightly.

Moreover, there is a close and more satisfactory fitting of the socket, with the weight-bearing area situated at a point midway between the lower edge of the patella and the superior edge of the tibial tubercle, thus preventing all pressure on any bony prominences. The limb is easy to apply and to activate.

There are two primary factors which are essential if the patient is to become proficient at using the P.T.B. limb, and perhaps the more important of these lies in the hands of the therapist.

First, a well-fitting socket is essential. This is the responsibility of the prosthetist, but correct fitting will not alone produce satisfactory results. It must be accompanied by good, strong quadriceps action. This is the responsibility of the therapist. Before limb-fitting, weight-resisted exercises instituted at the appropriate time are essential for all below-knee amputees and may have to be continued during

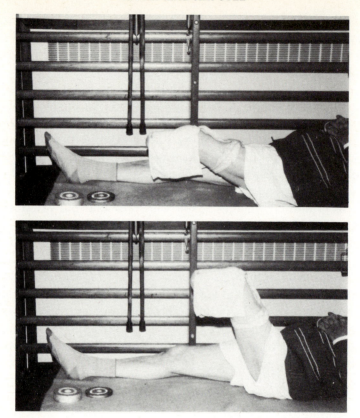

Fig. 34 and 35.    Resisted quadriceps exercises for the below-knee amputee.

prosthetic training and at home. For this purpose the following method is suggested.

Fix a weight bag to the stump with the patient lying supine. Start with a static contraction of the quadriceps group, then concentric hip flexion for straight leg raising. When the stump is approximately 10 cm (4 in) off the ground begin eccentric work of quadriceps until the hip and knee joints are at rightangles. Stop the movement and prepare to lower the thigh and stump; as the thigh is lowered there is concentric muscle work of the quadriceps to reach the ground in a state of static contraction. Follow with a short relaxation of all muscles and give 100 repetitions in sets of ten, increasing the weights accordingly.

*Requirements.* Wallet-type weight bag with loop. Above-knee fixing strap. Variable weights (Figs 34–35).

UNILATERAL SYME'S AMPUTEE

Prosthetic training for the Syme's amputee is not difficult for the patient or the therapist, provided that the pre-prosthetic phases of treatment have been given with an understanding towards limb-wearing. The most important question at this stage is what *type* of Syme's amputation is one dealing with? Is it classical or modified? Previous information given on p. 4 will clearly indicate possible complications.

*Application of Limb.* There are three important points that need careful observation when applying a Syme's prosthesis: (1) check that the stump sock has been pulled well up covering the distal end of stump smoothly; (2) check that the distal end of stump is resting directly over the centre of the weight-bearing pad of the limb; (3) check that the limb is securely fixed to the stump; if the limb is loosely applied it will slip up and down as the patient is walking, causing stump damage.

If the amputation is the modified Syme's then the therapist should check with the limb-fitting medical officer as to whether the patient's stump is full end-bearing or partial weight-bearing on the condyles of tibia.

With the limb correctly applied the patient will only need to become accustomed to the limb before a good walking pattern is achieved. Crutches, walking frames tripods etc. should not be used with this level of amputation. Any complaint from the patient of pain at the distal end of the stump should be reported to the limb-fitting medical officer, it would be a mistake to encourage these patients to weight-bear on their hands through a walking aid.

*Functional Activities.* Only one feature needs to be remembered during the teaching of functional activities. Situations such as stair climbing or negotiating the single step, whereby the patient may attempt to put just the foot on to the step, as normal, must now be corrected by placing the heel of the amputated foot well on to the step and extending the knee.

# 14

# Basic Principles of Prosthetic Training

## UNILATERAL BELOW-KNEE

It would be easy to believe that the walking training of the single below-knee amputee is a little less important than that of the above-knee amputee because, it is said, the patient having a knee joint should find it a more simple process.

This, however, is untrue; certainly the below-knee amputee should do better because he has an advantage with regard to the site of amputation. It will be found, when taking all things into account, that it is as difficult for a below-knee amputee to get accustomed to his artificial limb as it is for any other amputee.

It should also be stated that the below-knee stump is the most likely to break down during prosthetic training. The causes for this are few, but the one which is probably of most frequent occurrence is the incorrect method used by the patient when putting on the limb. The therapist can play a large part in preventing such a breakdown by rigidly checking the application of the artificial limb and making sure that the patient understands the importance of following the rules which apply to his particular prosthesis.

If the downward thrust of the stump into the socket is not maintained while lacing up the corset, the stump will be held out of the socket, resulting in friction at the lower end of tibia or just below the tibial tubercle.

In the case of short stumps, however, this method does not always prevent friction from taking place, and sometimes the short stump continues to come out of the socket during flexion. To overcome this a cross-knee strap can be attached to the metal uprights of the corset just above the knee joint. This strap will assist in maintaining the downward thrust of the stump into the socket. It should be noted that if the strap is drawn too tight it will to some extent restrict the movement of the knee.

## PYLON

It is not uncommon to find that the primary prosthesis issued to the below-knee amputee is an above-knee type of pylon, with the below-knee stump fitting into a soft leather or felt socket which is situated between the uprights. The socket can be made from metal or leather with adjustable corset (Fig. 21). The technique of training used in these cases is the same as that for the above-knee pylon. It must be remembered, however, that the below-knee stump must be exercised frequently in extension and flexion and that *while wearing the pylon the stump remains bandaged.*

This type of prosthesis is supplied to enable the patient to become ambulant early, before measurements are taken for the permanent below-knee limb. If the pylon has the leather adjustable socket, it is important to buckle up the strap and buckle at the top of the corset before lacing the corset. If this is not done, weight-bearing may well be taken on the distal end of stump, and not on the ischial tuberosity.

## PERMANENT BELOW-KNEE PROSTHESIS (WITH KNEE LOCK)

In some instances the limb medical officer may consider that the below-knee stump will not tolerate the normal functions of the permanent prosthesis, and so he may order a ring catch joint to be fitted, thus making it a permanently stiff knee joint while walking and yet at the same time permitting flexion of the knee when sitting. This ring catch joint may be hand-operated or semi-automatic.

For this type of prosthesis the techniques of training are as for the above-knee, with knee lock.

## BELOW-KNEE LIMB WITH NO LOCK

Where there is no lock attached, walking training follows the same lines as for the above-knee amputee with articulated knee joint, i.e. (a) standing balance; (b) knee flexion control; (c) single step taking; (d) free walking; (e) functional activities.

## PATELLA TENDON-BEARING LIMB

With this limb all patients will no doubt experience some difficulty in getting used to the new position of the stump. A large percentage of established below-knee amputees who have changed over from the corset type to this limb prefer it, especially once they have got used to the absence of the corset.

However, of the new primary below-knee amputees with stumps who are not yet fully established and are starting prosthetic training on the P.T.B. limb, it will be noticed that unless care is taken these patients will quickly develop a poor gait and frequent stump damage. To overcome these problems the following observations should be made during the early periods of training.

The stump sock should be pulled well up over the edge of the socket. The cuff suspension should be comfortably tight to support the limb, but should not restrict the joint movement or cause any pinching of the tissues. With some female patients it may be found that instead of the cuff suspension an elastic stocking is used. This should be firmly fixed to a suspender belt front and back. A loosely applied limb will give rise to excess piston action of the stump within the socket, making the patient feel insecure and possibly causing stump damage.

With the limb correctly applied, and the patient standing between the walking rails, teach the following:

1. Basic balance exercises followed by alternate knee raising, with the opposite hand holding on to the rail or stick. This will encourage early and full weight-bearing on the limb.

2. Flexion of the hip of the amputated side, followed by knee flexion and extension. It is important that the patient fully understands that the stump must flex and extend the limb.

3. Free walking between the rails, observing the length of pace and a normal swing phase from the knee. Short steps should be encouraged at first (if long steps are permitted a limping gait will follow). Any evidence of genu valgum on the amputated side should be reported early to the limb medical officer. It is not advisable to continue with prosthetic training until the alignment of the limb has been checked by the prosthetist.

Because the socket has been set in some slight degree of flexion, the patient is inclined to place the foot of his artificial limb down flat on to the ground as he steps forward. This tends to lead to stump damage and a limping gait if not corrected. Should the patient complain of pain at the distal end of tibia, or around the tibial tubercle, it will be found that the lower limb is being allowed to swing forward from the hip joint with little or no movement from the knee joint, and the foot being placed flat down on to the ground. The whole pattern of walking is incorrect.

To overcome this have the patient stand with the artificial limb to the rear and weight-bearing. Instruct the patient to transfer his body weight on to the sound limb. The heel of the artificial foot should now be raised off the ground, the knee slightly flexed and the toe remaining on the ground. The quadriceps now work concentrically to extend the knee and carry the limb forward, the heel being placed down just in front of the sound limb. The quadriceps now work statically for a brief moment holding the knee in extension. Then, as the body weight passes over the limb the quadriceps work eccentrically, flexing the knee. This should be repeated until the patient is fully conversant with what is required. Short periods of walking should be encouraged and the stump should be examined at frequent intervals.

During rest periods of sitting the patient may still complain of pain at the distal end of tibia, this being most painful when standing up. If the patient is asked to demonstrate it will be seen that he has been sitting with his knee joint flexed at a full 90°, if not more, and is attempting to stand up on to a flexed knee. The remedy lies in instructing the patient to sit with his knee slightly extended and, on standing up, to press up with the sound limb, drawing the artificial limb backwards at the same time to weight-bearing when the limb is extended. This will prevent any friction or pressure from taking place on the tip of tibia. At a later date when the stump has hardened up to the limb, a more normal sitting position can be adopted.

FUNCTIONAL ACTIVITIES

Functional activities for the unilateral below-knee amputee, with the exception of stair climbing, are the same as those for the above-knee amputee as described in Chapter 12.

STAIR CLIMBING, UNILATERAL BELOW-KNEE

Most below-knee amputees are able to climb stairs in the normal manner; some, however, will complain that stair climbing causes the stump to become painful. The greatest offender is the patient who attempts this activity too soon in his programme without the use of hand rails. Very few people with two sound legs go up and

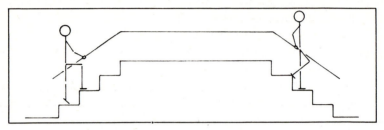

Fig. 36.    Unilateral below-knee amputee negotiating stairs. Note position of the feet.

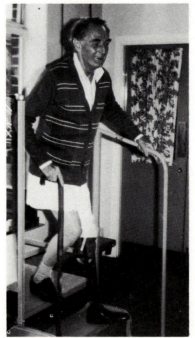

Fig. 37.    Amputee with below-knee patella tendon pylon descending stairs with one stick and handrail. Note position of the pylon foot over the edge of step tread and the stick on the same level as the pylon.

down stairs without using a handrail, so why should amputees be expected to do so in the first week or so of their training?

When teaching this activity the following method is suggested. Teach the patient to go up by placing the whole of the artificial foot on to the step. By bracing the knee into extension, and being assisted by the drive of the sound leg as the foot goes into plantar flexion, the body will be raised with little or no pain on the anterior aspect of stump. High steps should at first be avoided because attempts to go up these will only develop a hopping action.

When descending stairs it is advisable to place only the heel of the artificial foot on the step, with the foot well over the tread of the step (Figs 36–37). This will allow easy flexion at the knee joint.

Until the stump hardens a little, this activity will cause a little discomfort; therefore it is wise not to press the issue too much at the beginning.

## STICKS

As was explained earlier, it is easy to expect the unilateral below-knee amputee to progress much more quickly than those with amputations at other sites. In some respects this may well be true, but it is not true to assume that because the patient has a below-knee amputation he should discard his sticks much sooner than an above-knee amputee. Many amputees are still using sticks after many months of limb wearing and it will be found that many of them are doing so simply because they had their sticks taken away too soon during their prosthetic training periods; in consequence they failed to gain self-confidence.

The problem of using sticks is indeed a psychological one for the patient, and demands respect from the therapist. Often sticks are used as props, and this is due only to the lack of progressive balancing exercises in the early days, which had been omitted because the patient was a below-knee amputee.

## THE SLIDING SOCKET

The sliding socket is moulded to a plaster cast of the stump, thus giving a closely fitting leather socket, and it remains in contact with the stump. During walking the socket and the stump together make a piston-like movement within the metal container. It may only be a very slight movement but it is present; therefore, this sliding socket will prevent friction taking place on the stump and will also give the patient the reassuring feeling that the limb is securely fixed and is a part of him.

It is sometimes stated by the patient that he feels the limb is falling off when he lifts it off the ground. This is generally the result of two things:

1. The limb has not been applied correctly
2. The socket and the stump together are not making the piston-like movements within the shin piece

The correction of (1) is simple; the correction of (2), should it be necessary, is for the prosthetist. He can, with permission from the limb medical officer, add to the socket a four-point elastic pick-up, which is attached to the socket and corset anteriorly and posteriorly. This will ensure a constant contact of stump and socket.

It may now be asked what happens when patients are fitted with an all-wood limb where there is no sliding socket.

Wood limbs are mainly issued to patients with below-knee stumps which are longer than the usual (10–14 cm), and it has been found that the long stump and the all-wood limb are best suited. It should not be considered, however, that this combination is essential, because sometimes it may be found that the long stump has been fitted with a leather socket with a metal limb.

The all-wood limb is also issued to patients with the ideal length of stump. These patients, it will be found, are either working in a very hot atmosphere or living in a hot climate. The wood will absorb any excess perspiration and eventually dry out, whereas the leather socket may tend to soften with perspiration and lose its shape when it finally dries out and hardens overnight.

However, should patients wearing the all-wood limb complain of friction on the stump, the circumstances should be reported to the limb medical officer (having first checked that the limb has been correctly applied). The patient would then be referred to the prosthetist for any necessary adjustment.

LEATHER BACK CHECK STRAP

The leather back check strap is attached posteriorly from the corset to the lower limb. Its aim is to prevent hyperextension of the knee joint.

With long use of the below-knee prosthesis, it is possible that the check strap has stretched, giving rise to some slight hyperextension—consequently the patient will complain of pain within the knee joint. Also, if the leather strap becomes stretched a clapping sound may be heard as the patient walks. Alternatively, it is not uncommon to find that the strap has contracted, becoming very tight and so preventing full extension; this will be easily noticeable. In both instances, a small adjustment is necessary to obtain a good, normal gait.

Finally, complaints are often made that the limb is pinching the tissues behind the knee when the patient flexes his knee. The cause of this is that some oedematous tissue is still present in this area and is being pinched between the lower posterior edge of the corset and the upper edge of the socket. This oedema may well subside, and it would be unwise, therefore, to make any immediate adjustment; if, however, this condition persists, an adjustment will have to be made.

## BILATERAL ABOVE-KNEE AMPUTEE

### ROCKER PEGS

Most bilateral above-knee amputees are issued with a pair of rocker peg prostheses (Fig. 38). These may be temporary or permanent, depending entirely on the decision of the limb-fitting medical officer.

The base of the rocker pegs are part of a circle, the radius of which is the distance from the ischial tuberosity to the ground. This ensures that when the rocker pegs are being worn in the erect position, the body weight is always directly over a point of contact with the ground. The patient is thus never off-balance, regardless of any hip flexion deformity accommodated in the sockets.

The height of the pegs is normally 45 cm (18 in) but it is a practice to increase the height to 55–60 cm as the patient progresses.

The pelvic band is joined together at the back, either by a lace or strap and buckle. This enables the patient to put the limbs on individually or as a pair.

## SOCKETS

Sockets are made from a light metal. The fitting and problems arising from these are the same as those for single above-knee amputees.

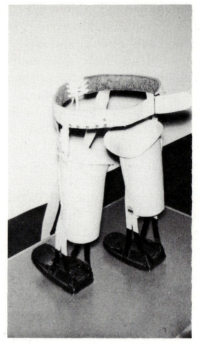

Fig. 38.    Bilateral above-knee rocker pegs.

The sockets will be set to accommodate any existing degree of hip flexion deformity. The greater the degree of flexion, the more diffi-cult it becomes to use the prosthesis; it can at times result in the inability of the patient to manage full-length articulated limbs, hence the importance of giving intensive stump exercises at the earliest possible time.

## APPENDAGES

Appendages consist of two shoulder straps which are crossed and sewn at the back, passing over each shoulder and clipping on to the pelvic band front and back. As previously explained, these should not be tight.

## TECHNIQUE OF APPLYING ROCKER PEGS

It is necessary to know that when rocker pegs are being applied, particularly if the patient is putting them on separately, correct adjustment of the pelvic band is most important to ensure correct fitting. To outline this clearly it should be explained that one of two methods is generally used by patients at home when applying artificial limbs: lying on the bed or sitting in a chair. In both these positions the rocker pegs can be applied separately or joined together.

When patients first take delivery of their rocker pegs, the adjustment of the lace, or strap and buckle, is set by the prosthetist and should remain as they have been set. Many patients, however, find it difficult to put on the limbs while they are joined together. They therefore separate the limbs and put them on one at a time.

The question now is: how do they adjust the back lacing etc? The answer is that this is invariably done by another member of the family or by a community nurse. Consequently the lace, or strap and buckle, may be too tight or too loose. Whichever is the case, the tuber seatings provided on the limbs are not supporting the ischial tuberosity. The rocker bases are either internally or externally rotated. This will cause a great deal of discomfort and slow down progress.

Some thought must also be given to the fact that some patients on rocker pegs will eventually progress to full-length articulated limbs. To apply long legs while sitting in a chair at home is very difficult and calls for a great deal of effort. It is necessary, therefore, to teach all bilateral above-knee amputees a method which is suitable for both types of prosthesis and one which is safe and practical. For these requirements the following method is taught. The patient begins by sitting on the bed. The limbs are laid out in front of him. Stump socks are put on and pulled well up. He then moves forward to sit over the pelvic band, with the stumps entering the sockets. It is here that difficulty is found in getting over the laced part of the pelvic band, but with practice and perseverance the patient soon learns to lift himself over this obstacle and to place his stumps well into the sockets.

Taking hold of both metal uprights of the pelvic band (one in each hand), the patient now takes the supine position and pulls the limbs further on to the stumps. Buckling the pelvic band loosely in front and rolling first to one side and then the other, he pulls up the pelvic band at the back and buckles it firmly in front. Finally, he pulls up the stump socks and rolls them over the edges of the sockets.

To get off the bed the patient needs to roll into the prone position and allow his limbs to slide down to the ground, pushing upright with his hands on the bed. Any further adjustments can be made when he has gained his balance.

It may be thought that this method would seem to be easier said than done; but it is safe, it is possible and, most important, it is suitable for both rocker pegs and full-length limbs. This procedure occasionally takes some patients a full hour at first attempt, but with practice it can be completed in 15 minutes or less, depending on the age and general condition of the patient.

The second method would appear to be a more suitable way (to slide off a chair into the rocker pegs), but in the case of long articulated limbs, which would stand much higher than the level of the stumps and would be capable of bending at the knee joint, this method is not very safe.

In any amputee unit, however, where there are walking rails between which the chair can be placed, the chair method is undoubtedly the quicker one to use. Consideration must be given, however, to the home circumstances of all patients. It would be pointless to teach any patient how to use his prostheses if it were not possible for him to put them on at home.

# 15

# Technique of Training— Rocker Pegs

The training techniques to be adopted depend much on the general condition of the patient. Some will have had previous experience of one artificial limb, others will be apprehensive about how they will manage. They need to have faith and confidence in the therapist on whom they are largely dependent at this early stage.

It is important, therefore, that understanding and patience are shown, particularly in dealing with the older patient and with those who are burdened with the added misfortunes of angina, arthritis, blindness or deafness; these are but a few of the complications that may be found in this group of patients.

The following sequence of training has been found to produce a satisfactory result within a period of four to six weeks. It is, of course, necessary to make adjustments to suit the needs of the individual.

*First Week.* Patient in rails; check fitting, then teach the following:
1. Standing balance
2. Hip updrawing, with full weight-bearing on opposite limb
3. Alternate single leg swinging forward and backward
4. Free walking exercise between rails

*Second Week.* Follow the pattern of the first week, with the following additions:
1. Introduce one stick and four-point walking
2. Watch carefully for circumducted gait
3. Free walking in the rails with one stick (which changes hands alternately)

It is at this stage that assessment can be made as to whether or not the patient will be able to manage sticks. If the situation appears at all doubtful it is best to introduce the tetrapod or tripod walking appliance immediately for early ambulation.

*Third Week.* Four-point walking out of rails, with sticks or walking appliance, accompanied by the therapist until the patient is able to go alone.

The remainder of the prosthetic training period is given to continued free walking practice and functional activities, i.e. sitting on to a chair; sitting down on the floor and getting up; stair-climbing; negotiating one step without rails (pavements etc.).

A point which may well be put forward is that to keep the patient in the rails for two weeks is perhaps a little too long before letting him move out into the open spaces. However, if the patient shows promise of doing well within the first two or three days he should be allowed out. In some instances a little longer time within the rails may be worth while, particularly if it means that the patient will finally be able to use sticks comfortably when he eventually ventures out into open spaces.

Age, general condition and intelligence must be the guiding factors, and since most of the rocker peg patients are elderly a little extra time is always well spent. Also worth mentioning is the fact that any patients discharged from the amputee unit on tetrapods or tripods are unlikely to become candidates for *long* legs. It is surprising how many elderly patients insist on attempting to try and wear full-length limbs. In view of this it is reasonable to allow the patient a little more time in the rails to appreciate one of the hazards of limb wearing at an early date, and so perhaps save a bitter disappointment later.

The most common problems arising during prosthetic training on rocker pegs are: (1) increased flexion contracture of hips; (2) increase or shrinkage of stumps; (3) pinching of tissues as patient sits down; (4) internal or external rotation of the rocker bases. These four problems have been discussed, as have the means of overcoming them. Either (1) or (2) may well be the cause of (3) and (4).

# 16

# Technique of Functional Activities—Rocker Pegs

Before going into the details of functional activities it should be pointed out that most rocker peg wearers are likely to be elderly patients; the aim, therefore, should be to spend a little more time in order to save energy and prevent fatigue. With this in mind some techniques less tiring than others are described.

### SITTING DOWN ON A CHAIR

The young or fit amputee wearing double rockers finds little difficulty in managing to sit down on a chair, provided it is not too high. It is far better to give others a set pattern to follow. They should approach the chair at an angle, the nearer leg being placed forward and the nearer hand being placed on the seat or arm of the chair. Bearing the weight on the rear leg, the forward leg is raised, and with a slight pivot on the rear leg the patient can sit down.

The height of the chair is very important. Investigations show that the ideal height for rocker peg wearers is a chair which measures 40 cm (15.5 in) from the ground to the top edge of the seat. It is also necessary that the chair-back should be straight and as near to a right angle with the seat as possible; arm rests are also a great asset.

### STANDING UP FROM A CHAIR

For those who are young and fit this activity will be no problem; they will simply slide forward on to the edge of the chair until the rocker bases are resting on the ground and extend the hips, assisted by their hands, pushing forward from the armchair rests or chair seat.

For others the following method can be taught. The patient should slide forward to the edge of the chair turning slightly towards the side of the weakest stump, the hand of this side remains on the arm-chair rest or seat of the chair. A stick is taken in the other hand and placed on the ground in front of the rocker base which is resting on the ground. The patient then slowly pushes himself off the chair to weight-bear on the outside limb and stick until his body is off the chair. Still holding the chair, the inside limb is now carried back-wards into extension.When stable, the other stick is taken up and the balance regained before commencing to walk. It is advisable that in the first one or two attempts the therapist should stand behind the patient to give a little assistance by holding on to the metal upright joining the pelvic band to the limbs.

A point worth remembering is that the height of the chair will make this activity simple or difficult.

SITTING DOWN ON THE FLOOR

Not all patients will wish to sit down on the floor. Nevertheless, this procedure should be taught because some patients would sooner sit on the floor than in a chair, and most bilateral amputees have to perform some home chores sitting on the floor. This instruction also has the advantage of providing an opportunity of teaching patients how to get up following a fall.

*Sitting Down.* Place both sticks forward in one hand, forming a tri-angular base. Slide the free hand down the sticks to the ground. With both hands now weight-bearing on the ground, flex the elbow of the side with the stronger stump and rest on the forearm, roll over to the same side, and adopt the 'long sitting position'.

The stout and heavily built patient will find it more difficult and no doubt will complain that the front of the sockets digs into his groin. This does not call for adjustment; it is unfortunately one of the hazards of limb-wearing.

*Getting Up.* Roll into the prone position, push up with the hands to lean on one stick, and then on the other. Regain balance and walk off.

This can be a very strenuous activity for some patients, and dis-cretion must be used when teaching it.

### FALLING

When falling, most rocker peg wearers fall backwards, having lost their balance and having flexed their hips. Because of the short distance from the ground they need only concern themselves with protecting their heads. To do this, every patient wearing rocker pegs should be instructed to pull the chin in to the chest when falling backward, at the same time trying to allow the body to relax.

### STAIR-CLIMBING (TWO HANDRAILS)

Grasp both rails, one in each hand, place the limb with the stronger stump on the edge of the first step and pull with both arms, lifting the other limb on to the same step. This procedure is repeated with each step.

### DESCENDING STAIRS (TWO HANDRAILS)

With both hands on rails stand close to the edge of the top step, turn slightly to the side of the weaker stump. The stronger stump is lifted outwards and lowered down backwards on to the lower step, flexing the hip of the opposite side. This leg is then lowered on to the same step and the whole procedure is repeated until the last step is reached. Should the handrails not extend beyond the last step it will be necessary to use one stick in the hand of the side that is being lowered on to the floor.

### STAIR-CLIMBING (SINGLE HANDRAIL)

Stand facing the handrail, grasping it with both hands. The limb nearest the step is placed forward, weight-bearing on the rear limb. The forward leg is then raised on to the first step, the stump being braced well into the back of the socket. Pulling up strongly with both hands, the patient places the other leg on to the same step in the same position as before, i.e. behind the forward leg. Repeat the same procedure for each step.

### DESCENDING STAIRS (SINGLE HANDRAIL)

Stand close and upright to face the rail which is held firmly with both hands. The limb nearest to the step edge is lifted outward and lowered backward on to the lower step, flexing the opposite hip and extending the arms to bear weight on the rear leg. The forward leg is then lowered on to the same step.

The patient now pulls himself into the erect position, weight-bearing once more on to the forward limb so allowing the rear leg to be lowered once more. Many problems may arise in this activity, but as stair climbing is almost a necessity all possible methods must be tried.

One problem that often arises, particularly when there is only one handrail, is that the patients find that the backward section of the rocker bases may be a little too long when being lifted on to the step. With permission from the limb medical officer, these may be shortened.

### SINGLE STEP (NO HANDRAIL)

This might be considered as being the most difficult manœuvre for patients on rocker peg prostheses and in most cases it is best left out of the training programme during the early stages of limb wearing. However, many patients will have to overcome this obstacle at home and, if it is not possible to have any form of support fitted, the method taught is the same as for climbing the first step with one handrail, with the exception that support and leverage are maintained by the sticks.

It should be understood that the rocker peg prostheses are not reserved only for above-knee amputees. They are, in fact, supplied to patients whose bilateral sites of amputation are as follows: bilateral below-knee; bilateral through-knee (disarticulation); one above- and one below-knee; one above- and one through-knee; one below- and one through-knee. Whatever the case, should the patient be wearing the rocker peg type of limb the sequence of prosthetic training is as has been described.

# 17

# Prosthetic Training for Bilateral Above- and Below-knee Amputees

## FULL-LENGTH ARTICULATED LIMBS

With full-length articulated limbs two single above-knee limbs are joined together by the pelvic band. In general, these limbs are finished off shorter than the patient's normal height. The correct fitting and problems arising with these limbs and the method of applying them are the same as those for the single above-knee or rocker peg prostheses. All bilateral above-knee limbs will be fitted with one knee lock, usually found on the side with the shorter or weaker stump. It may be automatic or hand-operated. Should it be the latter, this will give some indication that the patient may possibly use both knees free at some later date. Nevertheless, whichever is the case, prosthetic training should begin with one knee locked.

Previous experience on any type of prosthesis is always an advantage to the patient, but many habits may have been formed; it is therefore best to disregard these and start again from the beginning.

### IMPORTANCE OF BALANCE

The first and most essential basis for patients starting prosthetic training in this group is a good free-standing balance, the feet being approximately 20–25 cm (8–10 in) apart.

Progress in walking is delayed and general posture becomes poor if a good free-standing balance is not achieved early. Flexion contracture of the hips is often a difficult obstacle. It has been explained that the rocker bases allow patients to lean back on to the extended backward section and still remain balanced, regardless of hip flexion. On full-length limbs this is not possible; the stumps must always be fully extended to prevent the knee joints from flexing.

The sockets of the limbs will have been set to accommodate any flexion deformity. Nevertheless, patients will still tend to flex the hips even further to ease the tension.

It will be seen then that this problem alone is quite sufficient for the patient to cope with, not to mention the extra height, the weight and the new walking action. It can be expected, then, with most bilateral above-knees on full-length limbs, that during the first week or two they will tend to weight-bear to some extent on the sticks.

*Use of Sticks.* The correct length of sticks is important. If they are too long the patient will soon learn to use them as props, correct balance will become even more difficult, the elbow joints will remain flexed, forearm muscles will become fatigued and there is always the possibility of a nerve palsy in the hand from excess pressure.

### FOUR-POINT WALKING

Four-point walking is next in importance. This method ensures that weight-bearing is distributed evenly on both limbs, it encourages an even pace, and is comparable with the natural walking coordination of opposite arm and leg. It will take anything from three to six months of continual use before these patients become fully proficient and independent in the use of full-length articulated limbs.

### WALKING FAULTS

It is essential that the patient should feel secure in his limbs, and this brings to mind two things which can occur during the early days of training and which can cause the patient to become a little apprehensive. They should be looked for and are, fortunately, easily noted: pivoting on one or both heels; knee shoot of the free knee. These two problems may be seen together, but of the two pivoting is the more common. This occurs as follows:

When the limbs are in the walk-forward position and the patient attempts to weight-bear on to the forward limb, this tends to pivot into external rotation; in some instances the rear limb will do likewise. The free knee, whether it be forward or backward, may also tend to flex slightly (knee shoot). This is due either to hip flexion while walking or to slight hardness of the foot rubbers. To check this, stand the patient erect, bearing full weight evenly on both limbs. Grasp the foot of the suspect limb and attempt to move it into external and internal rotation. If the sole of the shoe is held firmly on the ground by correct weight-bearing with the body upright, this attempted movement will be difficult; it may then be assumed that the pivoting is caused by the patient's walking with some degree of hip flexion in excess of that which has been accommodated in the socket.

On the other hand, should it be found that while the patient is standing erect the sole of his shoe is raised slightly off the ground, thus making the attempted movement easy, this may well indicate that the foot rubbers are too hard. The prosthetist will soon put this right.

### THE TIME FACTOR

The bilateral above-knee amputee needs approximately four to six weeks to get fully accustomed to his new limbs and to gain the knowledge necessary at this stage. Until he has been at home for some weeks he will not know just how usefully his limbs will serve him.

### THE IMPORTANCE OF PHYSICAL FITNESS

It would be safe to say that only the young and fit amputees use the full-length limbs at home to their full advantage. The older patient invariably reverts to using his rocker pegs for mobility and to using the long legs only for short periods and for cosmetic reasons.

The main reason for this is the age and general physical condition of the patient. Here again the problem is that of physical incompetence, and this underlines the importance of general active exercises at the earliest possible opportunity. These are: warming-up classes to music, recreational therapy groups, encouragement for patients to wheel themselves about in their wheel chairs, weight-resisted exercises for the upper limbs, and swimming wherever possible. These are all excellent methods of helping to overcome this problem of physical failure.

## BALANCE

The average patient on full-length articulated limbs can usually manage to walk outside the rails within the first two weeks, but he will feel confident only with a good free-standing balance. It is therefore advisable that this should be achieved first; for this purpose the following sequence of training can be adopted:

*First Week.* The greater part of the first week is spent in the walking rails with one limb locked, practising the following:

1. Standing balance with the use of rails
2. Free-standing balance without the use of rails
3. Hip updrawing of locked limb with the use of rails
4. Knee flexion control of free knee with the use of rails
5. Transferring of weight from one limb to the other in the walk-forward position, alternating the forward limb

The remainder of the time is given to walking between the rails, introducing the four-point method, checking gait and posture.

*Second Week.* As above, using one stick and one hand on the rail, with the exception of free-standing balance where one stick only is used, the stick first in one hand then the other. After the second or third day introduce two sticks and repeat the whole procedure using the sticks in place of the rails.

If, at the end of two weeks, the patient is still unstable, it is usually more rewarding to allow more time in the rails. The length of time during which the patient is under instruction daily will, of course, play a great part in his progress. The above programme and those previously given are based on a two-hourly period each day for three days a week.

As soon as the patient is out of the rails and walking confidently, the next aim is to perfect functional activities in the following order:

1. Sitting down and rising from a chair
2. Turning while walking
3. Stair-climbing
4. Negotiating one step without rail
5. Walking backwards and sideways

6. Falling and rising from the floor
7. Picking up small objects from floor
8. Walking up an incline

## BILATERAL BELOW-KNEE AMPUTEES

The technique of prosthetic training for the double below-knee amputee should be based on the method given for the single below-knee amputee, working on each leg alternately when in the rails, with additional attention being given to free-standing balance, four-point walking and a constant checking of the application of limbs when applied by the patient.

Strong quadriceps action is essential if the patient is to do well. Where this is lacking, or where the stump is short, it may be necessary to fit a ring catch joint to one leg to stabilize the joint for early ambulation; this decision must be made by the limb-fitting medical officer.

### STICKS

Again beware of the patient tending to discard one or both sticks too soon; this can easily be the cause of damage to the stumps. The point at which patients are ready to dispose of one stick will become evident. This is usually when they have acquired a confident free-standing balance.

# 18

# Functional Activities for Bilateral Above-knee Amputees

## FULL-LENGTH ARTICULATED LIMBS

### SITTING DOWN ON A CHAIR

This can become a major problem with some patients and care must be taken to see that the instructions given are clearly understood before they attempt to sit on or rise from a chair.

Strong upper limbs, good balance and coordination are the main assets. Complications such as arthritis of the hands and arms, the use of spinal supports, paresis of the upper limbs, blindness or the absence of one arm will add to the difficulties. It may even be necessary to have fixed appliances on the wall or overhead to enable the patient to achieve his object.

There is one method which is safe and easy to accomplish for the average patient. Let him approach the chair from an angle, with the unlocked knee nearest to the chair and placed forward. Full weight-bearing is then taken on the rear leg, which remains locked. The nearer hand is placed on the seat or arm of the chair and the body weight is now distributed between this hand and the locked limb. One stick is held in the other hand and placed *in front* of the locked limb; when stable, the unlocked knee is flexed slowly. The patient then pivots on the heel of the locked limb and lowers his body into the chair by slowly flexing the elbow of the weight-bearing arm.

No doubt, during the first few attempts, the patient will sit down rather heavily as the locked limb finally comes off the ground, but this disadvantage will soon be eliminated with practice.

### RISING FROM A CHAIR

One limb is locked and the heel rests on the floor. The patient turns slightly towards the free knee side; the hand on this side is placed on the seat or arm of the chair and the stick in the other hand is placed *in front* of the locked limb.

A coordinated movement of hip extension on the locked limb and pressing up with the hand on the chair will result in the patient standing with a three-point triangular base with one hand still resting on the chair. The unlocked knee is stabilized by bracing the stump in extension before removing the hand from the chair and taking up the second stick and positioning the feet for walking.

It is advisable to give a little assistance at the first few attempts by taking hold of the metal upright of the pelvic band on the locked side so as to help the patient to raise himself as he presses upwards. The amount of pressure on the stick must be minimal because too much pressure will offer resistance to the body being raised out of the chair.

This method can be achieved in a relatively small space, and once mastered it is far less cumbersome than any other known method. However, there is no hard and fast rule: each patient is an individual and must be treated as such.

### TURNING WHILE WALKING

When walking outside the rails, most patients tend to walk from one chair to another in preference to turning round and walking back to their own chair. This is sometimes due to the fact that they are apprehensive of making the turn.

To simplify this the following instructions can be given. If the patient wishes to turn left he should pause for a moment with his right leg forward and on the ground. He pivots slightly to the left and takes two more steps; when the right foot is again forward he repeats the pivot, and so on, until he is fully facing the opposite direction. It is necessary that this series of pivots should be taken through a half circle, and no attempt should be made to pivot completely round on the spot. Once these movements have been mastered with balance control, the patient will soon manage to turn round without stopping—by taking shorter steps with the inside leg.

### STAIR-CLIMBING

The basic pattern for stair-climbing is the same as that suggested for the rocker pegs, with a reminder that the emphasis is placed on strong upper limbs and that the bending knee precedes the locked knee when going up, bracing the knee into extension before pulling up with the arms. When coming down, the locked knee precedes the bending knee, the foot of the bending knee having first been placed over the edge of the step and the weight being borne on the hands while lowering the leg on to the step (Fig. 39).

It may well be possible to teach the more advanced patient to climb stairs with one handrail and one stick; which side the stick should be is a matter for experiment. It would, however, be advisable to begin with the stick on the locked limb side. (This, of course, can only apply where there are two handrails or the single rail is on the free-knee side.)

### NEGOTIATING ONE STEP WITHOUT RAILS (PAVEMENTS ETC.)

As with rocker pegs, mounting a step without rails is a difficult manœuvre, but it may be a little easier because of the extra leverage of long legs. The stronger patient may well be able to walk straight up to the pavement, place one instep on the edge and, with momentum and powerful hip extension, manage to overcome this problem. Others will need to approach the pavement from the bending knee side, swing the leg forward and upward on to the step, extend the knee and hip strongly, weight-bear with the stick on the lower level and lift the rear leg on to the step behind the forward limb.

Strong stumps, good balance control and coordination are essential (Figs 40, 41).

### WALKING SIDEWAYS AND BACKWARDS

Sideways and backwards walking need no explanation other than to say it is always worth while including these movements in the programme of prosthetic training because it is an advantage to the patient to be able to move sideways and backwards on his artificial limbs with confidence.

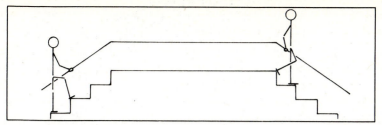

Fig. 39. Bilateral above-knee amputee negotiating stairs. Note position of the bending knee before its full extension, before pulling up with arms.

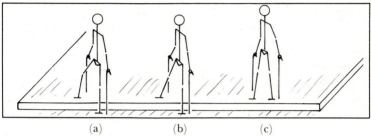

(a)          (b)          (c)

Fig. 40 Bilateral above-knee amputee negotiating a single step without hand rails.
*Going up*: (a) phase 1; (b) phase 2; (c) phase 3
*Coming down*: (c) phase 1; (b) phase 2; (a) phase 3

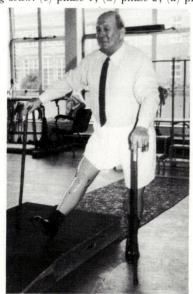

Fig. 41. Bilateral above-knee amputee negotiating a single step with no hand rail. Height of step 12–13 cm.

FALLING

The only instruction that can be offered under this heading is that of telling patients to try to relax as they fall and to encourage them to try falling on to a mattress. It will be seen that the patient will quickly flex at the hips and fall forward on to his hands. This seldom happens in a genuine fall, and mention must be made here of some of the situations which, if care is not taken, may well result in the patient finding himself on the floor.

When rising from a chair it is easy for the patient to fall if he takes his hand off the chair before the knee has been fully extended or if he presses too hard on to the stick. It is also possible that the locked limb will slip forward if the stump is not continuously braced back. In these instances the fall will be backwards.

If patients are wearing sorbo- or sponge-rubber heeled shoes there is the tendency for the heel to rebound slightly when striking the ground, and in consequence the knee joint becomes unstable for a short period. If reflex action is slow, as in the case of most elderly patients, they panic and fall, this time sideways towards the knee in question. This type of fall is typical in those patients who take short paces.

Another situation, and perhaps the worst, is a fall following a turn. The patient attempts to pivot too quickly on the inside leg without waiting until both feet are on the ground. This fall is usually backwards and sideways.

There are, of course, many other situations that result in the patient falling, many of them being accidental and unavoidable. However, those mentioned can be avoided by carefully observing the movements and warning the patient of possible dangers.

GETTING UP FROM THE FLOOR

Having made sure that all is well with the patient, the limbs should first be examined to make sure that all moving parts are functioning and are not damaged. The patient takes the long sitting position, locks one limb, gathers up his sticks, and places them on the bending knee side. He then rolls into the kneeling position on one knee, the locked limb extended backwards. The locked limb is then brought sideways into a widely abducted position, the weight being taken off the bent knee on to the hands and locked leg.

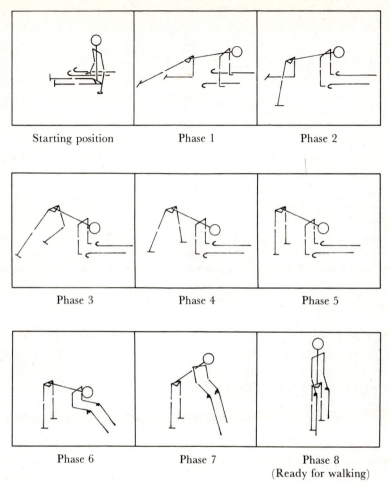

Starting position          Phase 1          Phase 2

Phase 3          Phase 4          Phase 5

Phase 6          Phase 7          Phase 8
(Ready for walking)

Fig. 42.    Bilateral above-knee amputee getting up from the floor.

The bending knee is then extended, with the hips rising upwards and backwards until even weight-bearing can be taken on both hands and legs with the hips flexed. The next move is to take one stick, place it forward and lean on it. When balanced, the patient takes up the other stick and again leans on both sticks. The trunk is slowly raised into an upright position, bringing one stick at a time closer to the feet. When the patient is fully upright, he positions his feet for walking off (Fig. 42).

It is advisable for the therapist to be standing nearby to assist if necessary during the last phase of the movement.

### WALKING UP AND DOWN AN INCLINE

To be successful in this the patient needs strong stumps with good extensor action. Short steps should be encouraged and a slight incline should be tackled first.

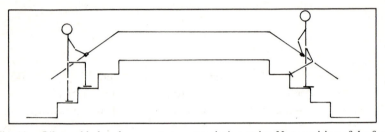

Fig. 43.    Bilateral below-knee amputee negotiating stairs. Note position of the feet.

## FUNCTIONAL ACTIVITIES—BILATERAL BELOW-KNEE

Patients in this category with one knee locked are taught functional activities as for the double above-knee with knee lock. Others with two free knees and strong stumps will no doubt find stair-climbing or getting up from the floor much easier, but a careful watch on the stumps must be kept because these activites, if begun too soon, will quickly damage them. Fig. 43.

# 19

# Other Prostheses

## THE TILTING-TABLE

The tilting-table type of prosthesis is used by patients with the following sites of amputation: (1) very short non-functional above-knee stumps; (2) disarticulation of hip joints; (3) hindquarter amputation (Figs 44–46).

The socket or bucket is made of light metal or blocked leather, with a padded seating area. Weight-bearing is on the ischial tuberosity of the amputated side in cases such as disarticulations and short non-functional stumps, and on the ischial tuberosity of the opposite side in cases of hindquarter amputation.

Just below the socket an automatic hip lock will be fitted which will lock the hip joint when extended and can be easily released for sitting down. There may or may not be a knee lock attached. By comparison with any other prosthesis, the tilting-table limb appears heavy and cumbersome. Patients, however, do remarkably well with them and it is often found that some patients with this limb become independent far more quickly than the normal above-knee limb wearer. A daily check on the scar tissue is necessary during the first week of limb wearing, and any friction or pressure points should be reported early to the limb-fitting medical officer.

### PROSTHETIC TRAINING

The action of walking for those with the tilting-table prosthesis is one of hip raising followed by a pelvic flick forward. As the limb follows the swing through to the forward position, the hip is lowered and the heel contacts the ground level with or just beyond the toe of the sound leg. Weight is then taken on the limb and the sound

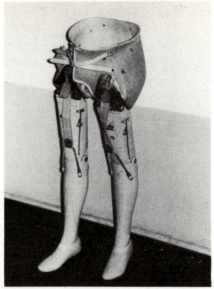

Fig. 44.    Through-hip permanent tilting-table prosthesis for a bilateral amputee.

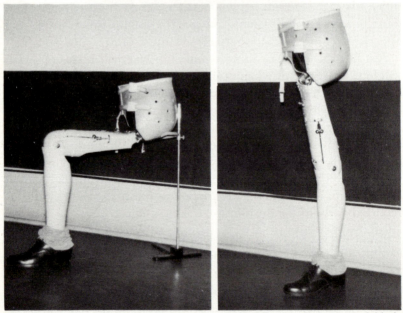

Figs 45 and 46.    Canadian type of prosthesis for hip disarticulation and hind-quarter amputation; incorporating mechanical hip flexion limiter (*left* sitting position; *right* standing position).

leg steps forward; short steps should be encouraged in the early days. With the hindquarter amputation where there is a great deal of muscle cutting, mobility of the hemipelvis must be adequate and strong to perform the pelvic flick. If this is not so, it will be found that patients will rise on to the toes of the sound leg in an attempt to prevent the toe of the artificial limb from striking the ground as it swings forward.

Free-standing balancing exercises are very important to these patients. It may well appear that they are evenly balanced on both limbs, but a closer look will reveal that most of the weight is being taken on the sound leg.

The application of this limb is best done in the standing position. No sock is worn, but instead the underpants or vest can be smoothly wrapped over the operation area. It is an advantage to know what article of clothing was used by the prosthetist when fitting the patient so that a correct application of the limb can be continued.

When the patient is comfortably settled in the socket, buckle up both straps, passing round the hips and waist. These need to be firm unless instructions have been given by the limb medical officer or prosthetist for the straps to be otherwise. There may be one shoulder strap that passes over the shoulder on the sound side.


## UNILATERAL THROUGH-KNEE (DISARTICULATION)

Patients with unilateral through-knee amputations have some advantage over the normal above-knee amputee as regards limb-wearing. There is a longer lever, a natural end-bearing surface on which full weight-bearing can be taken. Muscles acting on the hip joint are intact, providing a powerful stump, and problems of circulation are less frequent.

The limb may be made of an all-metal material with a pelvic band, or a leather thigh socket with distal end-bearing can be supplied, shaped snugly to the thigh over and around the bulbous distal end, with an anterior lacing division (Fig. 29).

Because of the length of stump no knee control unit can be fitted with this type of prosthesis. In the early days, therefore, the tendency for knee-shoot is obvious. It would appear that these patients find more difficulty in controlling knee-shoot than those with a normal above-knee stump. The instinctive habit to contract the quadriceps must be associated with hip extension before full stability of the artificial knee joint can be achieved; until the patient understands that only by bracing the stump back into the socket can he control knee flexion, knee-shoot will remain obvious.

In some cases the limb medical officer may consider it necessary to add a ring catch joint, thus stabilizing the knee for early and safe ambulation. This lock may be either semi-automatic or hand-operated.

## LONG FEMORAL STUMPS

For long femoral stumps, where full end-bearing is seldom satisfactory, the same types of limbs can be supplied but with an ischial seating area at the top of the corset or socket for partial or full ischial weight-bearing.

The technique of prosthetic training for the through-knee or long femoral stumps is the same as that for the above-knee amputee with or without a knee lock.

## BILATERAL AMPUTEE (ONE ABOVE- AND ONE BELOW-KNEE)

For bilateral amputees with one stump above and one below the knee, instructions as for the single above- and below-knee amputee should first be given alternately to each limb before combining the two in a four-point walking technique.

From the point of view of functional activities it will prove helpful if the below-knee limb is considered the master limb, as for single amputees. For example, when stair-climbing the patient should go up with the below-knee leading and come down with the above-knee leading. As with all bilateral amputees, free-standing balance is important and should be achieved before the patient is brought out of the walking rails.

Because of the different patterns of neuromuscular coordination required to activate each limb, and the different sense of weight-bearing, these patients tend to be a little slower in progress during the first week or two.

APPLICATION OF LIMBS

The application of limbs is again best done on the bed when the patient is at home, putting the below-knee limb on first and making sure that the stump is placed well into the socket.

The younger and fit patients may well prefer to sit in a chair, put the below-knee limb on first, stand, and put on the above-knee; good balance and strong quadriceps muscles are necessary for this method.

Problems other than those already discussed are those of neuro-muscular coordination.

# 20

# Care of the Stump and Prostheses

## CARE OF THE STUMP

All limb-fitting centres can supply the amputee with information on the care of the stump, but it is as well to include a few words on the subject.

It is the therapist's responsibility to ensure that the patient is fully aware of the importance of stump hygiene. It should be explained that the stump is the 'commander' and should therefore be given the greatest respect, care and attention. Any form of stump damage will only retard the patient's progress.

Stump bandaging and the correct application of the limb have been discussed, and are essential for stump care. Further suggestions of stump hygiene are as follows. When the limb is taken off at the end of the day, the stump should be washed in hot water with a suitable toilet soap, and then rinsed again in cold water. Not every patient will be able to tolerate the immediate change of water temperature, and they should therefore be encouraged to make a gradual change from hot to cold water, finishing off with a brisk rubbing with a bath towel.

Therapists will understand the physiological effect that this will have on the tissues. The patient, however, should be told why such shock treatment is suggested, and it takes only a few minutes of the therapist's time to explain this in simple language. This method of stump hygiene is indeed simple and inexpensive. It will, however, need to become a habit, involving time. Finding the time for stump hygiene must be considered one of the hazards of being an amputee, but it must be done. It is further recommended that with all levels of amputation where the patient is taking an ischial bearing prosthesis, washing should go up to and over the ischial tuberosity.

Stump socks should be changed every other day; in some cases where there is profuse perspiration the socks should be changed daily and washed regularly according to the instructions given on the official washing slip supplied by the Ministry.

It is not advisable to use any form of spirits on the stump to try to harden the tissues. This tends to dry up the skin and results in its becoming devitalized. Talcum powders should be used sparingly, if at all, when wearing the limb as this will tend to clog up the pores of the skin.

With some amputees, either wearing the P.T.B. limb or the suction socket limb, it is not uncommon to find that during the first few weeks of limb wearing the stump has perspired a great deal causing the patient some discomfort. Fortunately, this profuse sweating will subside as the stump becomes accustomed to being enclosed in the socket, but should it persist the following methods may be used to eliminate it.

The limb medical officer may order a small vent hole and a one-way valve to be put into the socket of the P.T.B. limb. This method, however, has a slight disadvantage in that there is the tendency for some patients to complain that the limb feels loose and as if it were falling off as they walk. This is an unnecessary distraction to the patient and to avoid this the limb medical officer may recommend the use of a simple antiperspirant solution. The stump can be treated once a day as necessary. Immediate results are not to be expected, but within ten days the profuse sweating should have subsided. It is not recommended that the antiperspirant solution be used continuously. If the condition has not cleared up within fourteen days the matter should be reported to the limb medical officer, and further advice will be given.

A further method can be employed to overcome this problem of stump care, and is used for all levels of amputation where it is found that skin irritation is holding up progress. The limb medical officer can supply a Rem-Daw protective sheath. This is a nylon undersock and is applied to the stump under the normal woollen stump sock. The use of oil or massage creams to massage the stump is not recommended. There are a few exceptional cases where there is adherent scar tissue around the suture line that may benefit from this treatment.

## CARE OF PROSTHESES

The artificial limb remains the property of the Ministry and it is unwise to attempt any form of repair or adjustment. Oiling, loose screws, broken appendages etc. should be dealt with by the limb makers, and any such need should be reported *early*.

The following procedure will help to keep the limb in a good, serviceable condition:

1. Each day after use the socket should be wiped with a clean damp cloth (not wet).
2. When the limb is not in use, and there is a knee lock fitted, it is advisable to lock the knee joint.
3. When storing the limb it should be wrapped up free from dust and kept in a dry place.
4. At all times keep the ankle and knee joints free from water.
5. If patients are in possession of a duplicate limb it is advisable that they should use each limb alternately. If the duplicate limb is not serviceable, the fact should *at once* be reported to the limb centre.

## BACK TO WORK

Many amputees who are still able to work are faced with the problem of how soon they can return to full employment and whether they can return to their previous jobs. The answer must depend on several factors—type of employment, site of amputation, cause of amputation, patient's psychological outlook towards limb wearing and if he is competent on his prosthesis.

To try to enlarge on this subject would take a great deal of space and it is not really within our province. But it must always be borne in mind that the primary aim is to endeavour to get all employees back to full time work as soon as possible.

During the pylon stage and at the end of prosthetic training the therapist may well be asked by the patient if he can return to work. This problem must be decided by the patient and his medical officer. Therapists should give encouragement at all times without committing themselves one way or the other.

In many cases compensation may be pending, and there may be contraindications to certain types of employment of which the therapist is unaware.

Those patients who are known to the therapist to be ready to return to work and who are capable of doing so can be referred to the visiting Disablement Resettlement Office (D.R.O.) or, in the few hospitals where one is employed, to the Hospital Resettlement Officer (H.R.O.), if any employment problems arise, before discharge from the amputee unit. It is not necessary for the patient to be unemployed; a change of job with his previous employer may still be possible, or a course of employment rehabilitation may be recommended under the employment service agency scheme.

## LIMB APPLIANCES AND ATTACHMENTS

Certain additional items can be prescribed by the limb medical officer to serve particular purposes. The following extras are available:

Buckle guards
Trouser and other clothing guards
Stocking guards (primarily for women)
Nylon braces in place of webbing where preferred
A device for varying the height of the heels of certain types of leg for ladies
Rubber socks for those engaged in wet occupations
Matt or flock finish on legs for ladies
Non-skid crampons for male amputees to prevent slipping on ice or snow

If it is thought that one of the above items might help the patient he should discuss this with his limb medical officer

## STUMP SOCKS

Woollen stump socks are supplied by the limb fitting centre and replaced, when necessary through wear and tear, on application to the limb centre.

With the exception of the hindquarter and the disarticulation of hip, all other levels of amputation will require stump socks. A supply of these will be given to the patient when taking delivery of the temporary pylon, and a further supply when taking delivery of the first permanent limb. Each patient will receive a selected stump sock specific to his or her stump size and the same size sock should be used at all times unless changed by the limb centre.

It is the therapist's responsibility to ensure that the patient understands the need to maintain a healthy stump and comfortable limb wearing by changing the stump sock every other day. The socks should be washed correctly in lukewarm water using a suitable washing powder for 'all wool' garments. Following washing, the socks should be laid flat on a towel and left to dry out. This method will help to preserve the socks and keep them soft for comfortable limb wearing. Stump socks should not be dried quickly by direct heat, nor should they be ironed dry. Socks that are not washed correctly—and frequently—become hard to the skin and may be the cause of friction soreness in the groin.

Unless otherwise stated, the limb socket is made to accommodate the stump and one stump sock only, the ischial tuberosity sitting on the ischial seating. Following exercise and walking, in most cases the stump is expected to reduce in size. This allows the stump to slip off the ischial seating into the socket causing much discomfort in the area of the adductor tendon or the ramus bone. When this occurs the therapist should advise the patient to use an extra sock. Should it become necessary for the patient to wear three or more socks for comfortable limb wearing the therapist should report this to the limb centre. Before doing so, however, it will be necessary to check that three socks or more are in fact needed, many patients in the early days of limb wearing would be very happy to wear more than the one sock as a means of easing the pressure off the ischial tuberosity. If this is allowed to take place the pylon will appear to be too long thus encouraging a circumducted gait, a habit difficult to eliminate.

# 21

# Special Cases

It is not uncommon to meet patients who have disabilities other than amputation. It might well be thought that patients with *epilepsy, cardiac incompetence, blindness, deafness, obesity, hemiplegia, spina bifida* or *amputation of the upper limb* would find the management of an artificial lower limb very difficult. Fortunately, this is not so. Many more complications arise from stumps that either have not had adequate physical treatment or have been badly bandaged. Amputees who fall into any of the above categories should, however, be considered as special cases and justify some further individual attention and care.

All amputees discussed here as special cases are assumed to be unilateral lower limb amputees, but should the therapist be required to treat bilateral amputees much additional thought and consideration will be needed to make them independently safe on their artificial limbs.

## THE EPILEPTIC AMPUTEE

Extra individual attention towards the epileptic amputee should not be made too obvious; the average epileptic patient strongly resents any implication that he is at all different from his fellow men. This resentment is silent, and the first indication that the therapist may have of it is when the patient fails to attend for treatment.

Prosthetic training for the epileptic amputee is the same as for any other amputee with the exception that the therapist should take care to see that the patient is in no danger of falling and he is not overstressed by excitement and enthusiasm. At the beginning of training the therapist should explain to the patient that he is fully aware of the problem, and that it will make no difference at all. It will be found that the patient's only concern will be 'what will those around me think, should I have a seizure?' If the patient's mind can be put at rest on this matter there should be no further need for sheltered treatment. Suitable exercises and group activities have not yet, in the author's experience, proved to be a contraindication to the epileptic amputee.

### CARDIAC INCOMPETENCE

Heart cases and patients suffering from hypertension tend to make good progress on artificial limbs provided that the therapist has graded and increased the patient's exercise tolerance with care. There should be no cause to hide from the patient the fact that he must take his time, and make progress slowly. Other than this the training programme is the same. It is in general more acceptable to the patient to appreciate for himself just how little, or how much, his condition will allow him to do on his artificial limb.

### THE BLIND AMPUTEE

The blind amputee will present the therapist with a problem of time and patience. This is particularly so if the patient is elderly and has only recently become blind. It is highly important that the blind amputee should have the opportunity of examining his pylon or permanent limb by his sense of touch so that he may become accustomed to his limb before attempting to use it.

The therapist should explain carefully each part of the limb, its purpose and how it will function. The blind amputee will be quick to learn and respect the therapist who expresses his understanding of the patient's problem in this way. It is time-consuming, but it should be carried out. It then becomes easier for the patient to discuss the limb and explain any discomfort or strangeness that he cannot see.

Prosthetic training for the blind is the same as for any other amputee, with the exception that the therapist should stay with the patient at all times until he is conversant with the locking mechanism of the limb. All instructions should be crystal clear and fully understood by the patient before being carried out. Emphasis must be placed on achieving a confident free-standing balance before attempting to walk. When the blind amputee is able to walk out of the rails with two sticks it will be seen that, if left alone, he will drift either to left or to right, but will seldom go in a straight line. This would indicate that the blind amputee should always be accompanied when walking out in the open spaces.

Concerning walking with a free-knee action, first consideration must always be given to the patient's safety. No attempt should be made at walking with a free-knee action until the patient is confident and conversant with his limb. When he is finally at home in familiar surroundings, he will move about more safely and confidently.

### THE DEAF AMPUTEE

The biggest percentage of deaf amputees are those who have lost their hearing due to senility. A smaller percentage are those who are deaf from birth and, in most instances, those of the latter group are also dumb.

The elderly deaf amputee needs a great deal of individual attention mainly due to the lack of good communication. This problem is sometimes eased by the use of hearing aids or sign language but the best known method of communication, regarding the deaf patient's training on his limb, is by demonstration. The therapist will need to be tolerant and understanding; he may need to repeat his demonstrations several times before the amputee understands what he is required to do. Frustration and failure will quickly develop from the therapist who grows impatient. An added advantage is for the deaf amputee to be able to watch other amputees of the same level of amputation walking. It is suprising how quickly he forms a mechanical appreciation of what is required and performs it himself. The techniques of prosthetic training do not alter; the most important factor is a good working relationship between the patient and therapist.

### THE OBESE AMPUTEE

The obese amputee presents two main difficulties.

1. The difficulty of achieving a satisfactory fitting.
2. The management of a continued correct application of the limb by the patient.

These two problems are due to an abundance of adipose tissue round the stump and abdomen.

There are, unfortunately, continued complaints of discomfort arising from the anterior superior aspect of the socket pressing into the lower abdomen. There is no justification in asking for the socket to be lowered in this region, as this would simply cause more tissue to roll out over the edge of the socket and be subjected to pinching when the patient sits, stands or walks. The use of abdominal corsets has been tried, but with only limited success.

The patient finds great difficulty in keeping the limb in a correct position; it ultimately assumes the inwardly rotated position, causing pressure in the groin and pinching of the tissue when weight-bearing on the limb.

It might well be thought that a larger socket would suffice but this only adds to the discomfort; the medial lip of the socket would come into contact with the scrotum or vulva. A further problem is that the excess body weight may well exceed the limited pressure tolerance of the tissues around the weight-bearing areas and result in skin abrasions, cysts and stump damage. The therapist is limited in his success with the obese amputee until the patient has succeeded in reducing his weight.

It must be stated, however, that the above comments do not apply to those amputees who are classified as obese but have good muscle function and are active.

### THE HEMIPLEGIC AMPUTEE

The amputee presenting hemiplegia would appear more difficult to rehabilitate on a prosthesis than he really is. So much of course depends on the severity of the cause, whether it was before or after amputation, which side is affected in relation to the amputation, and finally and most important the amount of recovery gained from the condition of hemiplegia. It is not within the scope of this book to discuss the physical programme for the hemiplegic patient but it is essential, from the prosthetic point of view, that the physical programme should be continuous and progressively intensive if the patient is to become successful on his limb.

Most hemiplegic amputees are those amputated some time after their cerebrovascular accident—the cause generally being vascular.

If the amputation is carried out on the same side as the affected arm, then the patient is likely to become ambulant a little sooner than one amputated on the opposite side. This is simply a matter of achievement of balance control.

During the pre-prosthetic phase of treatment special attention must be given to the sound leg and arm; the patient needs a great deal of practice in sitting and standing from a chair. It will be noticed that when the patient is attempting to perform these activities, plus standing balance, the shoulder and arm of the affected side tends to fall forward and inward towards the sound side, causing him to rotate his trunk, consequently making these activities difficult. Every attempt, therefore, should be made to train him to keep his shoulders square. The practice of putting the affected arm in a sling is a contraindication for the hemiplegic amputee. It is far more beneficial for standing balance, and walking on an artificial limb, if the amputee is taught to relax the arm and let it hang loosely by his side, not flexed and held across his chest. If trunk rotation, caused by the falling forward of the affected arm and shoulder, cannot be controlled, it may well lead to the patient's presenting a crab-like gait or possibly not being able to use his limb at all.

The amputee who has become a hemiplegic after amputation and has had some experience on a limb will have the added advantage of knowing how to manage his limb. Nevertheless, he will require the same individual attention, particularly from the psychological aspect. Being already aware of the problems of limb management he may now, having had a 'stroke', consider the task of using his limb too difficult. There will be of course the problems of putting the limb on. It is advisable to show a relative how this is done, but most amputees will manage alone after a short period of practice.

The techniques of prosthetic training for the hemiplegic amputee are the same. It might be found necessary for the stick to be used in the hand which is on the same side as the artificial limb. When this is so it is very important to ensure that the patient is not using the stick as a prop; the body weight must be taken on the limb, not the stick.

## THE SPINA BIFIDA AMPUTEE

Several cases of spina bifida are seldom seen in the limb-fitting centre. There are, however, some less severe cases that are seen from time to time. These patients are generally from the younger age group, having gone to the extreme of accepting amputation in the hope that they may become more mobile and independent in the future.

The supply and fitting of a prosthesis for the amputee in this category cannot be expected to be a simple matter. The therapist therefore who is responsible for the amputee's pre-prosthetic and prosthetic training must be prepared to give extra care in planning the patient's physical programme. Failure to succeed on a limb becomes a disappointment to all who have tried to make it possible, and in particular the patient.

The general approach to prosthetic training is the same given for whatever level of amputation is presented. The important problems are anaesthesia and weak muscles.

According to the severity of the spina bifida, varying degrees of diminished sensation can be found over a large, or small, area of the skin covering the stump and the buttocks. Most commonly affected is the area known as the 'saddle area' in which are situated two vital areas of limb fitting, the ischial tuberosity and the perineum. Some loss of sensation may also be found down the anterior and posterior aspects of the stump extending to the distal end.

Limb-wearing under these conditions can become critical if care is not taken. The prosthetist will make every effort to spread the body weight over a wide area to avoid any one place having to take the full load. During the early days of prosthetic training the therapist must frequently examine the stump and areas of anaesthesia, and any evidence of excess pressure must be reported early.

It would not be uncommon to find that the prosthesis supplied to the spina bifida amputee is not a standard one, but one that has been modified to suit the patient's requirements. The limb should be closely examined by the therapist to ensure that he is fully conversant with the suspension, weight-bearing areas and locking devices etc. Owing to the modification it may be found that the limb is now a little heavier than the standard limb, regardless of all the efforts made to keep it as light as possible.

Muscle weakness is also a common feature in the spina bifida amputee. The effort of limb wearing, therefore, can become very fatiguing and care should be taken to see that the patient does not do too much at the beginning. It has been said that the spina bifida amputee is one of the younger age group and very eager to make progress. This temptation to do just that little bit more too soon can produce muscle strain, or stump damage, and so delay the patient's progress.

### THE UPPER AND LOWER LIMB AMPUTEE

Not unlike the hemiplegic, rehabilitating the lower limb amputee with absence of the upper limb is not so difficult as it may at first appear. The most common type of combination seen in this category is the patient who has lost his upper limb in a road or industrial accident, followed some years later with the loss of his lower limb through vascular disease. With this type of patient the real problem is a psychological one of whether he will ever manage with the loss of two limbs. Every effort should be made, therefore, during the early days to convince the patient that with his cooperation and the will to succeed it is possible.

If the upper and lower limb amputations are on the same side the patient can be expected to make steady progress. It is, however, a little more difficult if the amputations are on opposite sides. This, as with the hemiplegic amputee, is a balance problem and the patient tends to take a little longer to become independently mobile.

The techniques of prosthetic training on the lower limb are the same. Some consideration, however, must be given to which hand the stick should be held in. At all times throughout the training on the lower limb the patient should be encouraged to wear his artificial arm; this helps considerably in gaining a good free-standing balance which should be achieved before attempting to walk. Should it be considered to use the stick in the artificial arm it must be remembered that it is more difficult to control. It would, therefore, be advisable to encourage the patient to use the stick in the sound hand, but if the sound hand is on the same side as the lower limb amputation care must be taken to see that the patient is not weight-bearing on the stick.

Should it be considered that two sticks would help the patient to become mobile, a walking stick appliance and adaptor can be supplied for the artificial arm. The handle of the stick is cut off, the cut end is fitted into the appliance, and the stick cut to the correct length. By means of the adaptor the stick appliance can be fitted into the rotary of the artificial arm, first removing the hand. The use of two sticks in this manner, however, is not always satisfactory for the above-elbow amputee as, apart from finding difficulty in controlling the stick movement, any weight-bearing on the stick will tend to move the arm socket upwards off the shoulder, thus causing pressure in the axilla. The below-elbow amputee is more able to use a stick in his artificial arm. In view of this slight complication the use of two sticks is an advantage for encouraging a standing balance, but the patient should persevere with one stick for walking, this being held in the sound hand. At the beginning, the patient will need help to apply his lower limb, but in due course he will manage alone.

# 22

# Special Cases—Bilateral Disarticulation of the Hip Joint

It could be difficult for the therapist to foresee what prosthetic possibilities lie ahead for the patient who unfortunately becomes an amputee necessitating bilateral disarticulation of the hip joints. It might well be thought that the patient would not walk again and that a life in a wheelchair would be all that would be possible after the sound healing of the amputated areas.

Fortunately this is not so. Amputees in this category will have passed through a limb-fitting centre and the younger and fit patient will have succeeded in reaching a reasonable limit of personal independence on artificial limbs. One thing is certain; such patients are not necessarily tied to a wheelchair existence. It cannot be considered an easy task; indeed, it is a very strenuous one and the therapist who fully appreciates the physical requirements can make it much easier for the patient. Furthermore, it must be considered that this responsibility lies with the therapist if these patients are to make the best of a difficult situation. For the elderly patient, and those presenting some contraindication to strenuous effort, then a wheelchair is no doubt the best solution.

PHYSICAL TREATMENT

At the earliest possible moment following amputation, if not before, the patient should start a full progressive physical programme of exercise and recreational therapy. This programme must aim at full mobility of the trunk and upper limbs through the medium of free exercises. Muscles of the upper limbs, shoulder girdles and the abdominal muscles should be treated by resisted exercises to reach a state of hypertrophy. Every aspect of physical medicine can be used in the pre-prosthetic programme for the amputee in this category. Much mechanical ingenuity is required in the making and fitting of prostheses of this kind and the success depends entirely on the physical condition of the patient.

### TYPE OF LIMBS

Two limbs of the tilting-table type (Figs 44–46) are fitted to the lower torso by a leather socket which embraces the pelvis. They are strapped together in front. The socket is fitted over the superior anterior crests of ilium; this has been found to be all that is necessary to secure the limbs adequately to the trunk. In some cases, however, shoulder braces may be fitted.

Weight-bearing is taken through the ischial tuberosity on both sides. The hip locks are automatic and will lock when the hip joints are extended. The knee locks are hand-operated. The hip flexion limiter is situated below the leather socket. This permits some slight movement of hip flexion, and controls the length of stride which can be adjusted to suit the patient's requirements.

### APPLICATION OF LIMBS

For the patient to achieve this alone, it is best managed on the bed. Some special article of clothing should be used to cover the amputated areas closely and smoothly. The limbs are laid out full length on the bed and the patient places his pelvis into the socket. When he is comfortable he should buckle up firmly, flex his hips, sit up and then fix shoulder straps, if fitted. A wheelchair is placed facing the bed, and the patient moves off the bed backwards into the chair. It should be remembered that if trousers are being worn, these should be put on and pulled over the socket before moving off the bed. As with any bilateral amputee the applying of his limbs is always a little difficult at the beginning. However, if the patient is active and physically fit he will quickly overcome this problem. A firm bed will make this task even easier.

### BASIC PRINCIPLES OF PROSTHETIC TRAINING

It is most important that the patient is conversant with the means of locking and unlocking the hip and knee joints, as failure to know this could result in his falling unexpectedly. The hip locks will become secure only when they are put into full extension; a slight click can be heard as the locks become engaged. It is well to train the patient to listen for this click. A release lever is found on the front of the thigh piece just below the socket for unlocking or fully flexing the hip joints. This lever will need to be pressed down and moved sideways into the holding slot, thus preventing the locking bar from springing back into the locking position. The joint then remains unlocked. During the first few attempts at unlocking the hip joints the locks may seem stiff and difficult to operate. In all probability the patient is tending to flex the hip joint before pressing the lever. By doing this tension is placed on the locking mechanism, thereby making it difficult to operate. The patient should be taught to extend the hip first.

The hand-operated knee-locks will need to be locked and unlocked manually; the operating plunger is found on the lateral aspect of the thigh piece. To lock the knee joint it must first be held in full extension, and the plunger then pressed inward and downward. To unlock the knee, the plunger is pressed inward and pulled upward. The patient may again find it difficult to operate. This is generally because the knee joint is not being held in its fullest range of extension while the plunger is being operated. The simplest and safest method of locking and unlocking the knee joint is with the patient sitting. Teach him to pull on the toes with one hand and operate the plunger with the other.

### BALANCE

Throughout this book balance exercises have been strongly stressed as being important factors for all amputees. For the bilateral amputee in this category a sound and confident free-standing balance is of the utmost importance. The patient who attempts to walk out of the walking rails without a good balance is unlikely to progress very far. Furthermore, a close examination of the socket will show that the upper edge is above the crest of ilium. Therefore, if the trunk is allowed to adopt a position of flexion by weight-bearing through the hands on to the walking aid, some pressure can be expected from the top of the socket which will affect the abdomen and the lower rib cage. This alone is sufficient evidence for the importance of a good erect free-standing balance.

A four-point walking pattern should be introduced as soon as possible, but no doubt the patient will prefer to start by placing both hands forward and then moving up to them. No hard and fast rule should be made about this; it is more important that the patient should first be able to establish the movement of his limbs. Progression to using sticks is possible finally, but should not be attempted until the patient has proved that he has a good and safe walking balance with the forearm crutches and is able to take full weight-bearing on his limbs. It is agreed that this method does not produce a normal gait, but most patients would prefer it to a wheelchair existence.

FUNCTIONAL ACTIVITIES

Common sense is the guiding factor in deciding what functional activities should be taught to the amputee in this category. The bilateral level of amputation and the necessary construction of the limbs do not lend themselves to making functional activities easy. It is suggested that activities such as sitting and standing from a chair should be taught. Negotiating steps and stairs with two handrails is possible but only if the patient has very strong upper limbs. Other activities such as getting up from the floor, picking up small objects from the floor, stepping over objects, walking up and down inclines etc. are extremely difficult and therefore not practicable to include as a routine factor in the programme.

STANDING UP FROM A CHAIR

This should be practised first between the walking rails. Teach the patient to lock both knee joints and disengage the locking bar from the flexion hold slot of the hip locks. Now instruct the patient to hold both rails and press up on to his hands. As his body is raised up out of the chair the hip-locks will extend and lock automatically. It must be understood that the movement is one of *pressing up*, not pulling up.

From this observation it can be seen that the simplest method would be to raise the height of the chair arm rests. With good balance, confidence and plenty of practice the patient will manage to stand from his chair with safety. The correct height of the arm rests will be determined by the height of the patient and the length of his arms. Detachable wooden arm rests are easily made and can be fitted to the chair when required or as permanent fixtures.

SITTING DOWN ON TO A CHAIR

This is a little more difficult because the hip-locks need to be operated manually to release the hip joints for flexion. The knee locks should be left locked until the patient is sitting. Teach him to manœuvre himself close to the chair, which must be very firm. The back of his limbs should touch the chair seat. Carefully dispose of the walking aids and put both hands backwards to rest on the arm rests. A sound balance must now be achieved on one limb. The hand of this side remains on the chair, while with the other hand the hip joint of the non-weight-bearing limb is unlocked by pressing the release lever downward and engaging it into the flexion hold slot. With both hands again resting on the chair the patient can now lower himself down on to the free hip side; the other hip joint can now be unlocked and the patient can take a more comfortable sitting position. Perfection of this activity can only come with practice, when the patient will manage to sit into his chair safely and smoothly.

These two activities are of vital importance to the patient if his limbs are to benefit him. He will, therefore, give the matter some thought himself and will no doubt offer suggestions of how he might manage to carry them out. Do not brush these suggestions aside; they should all be tried with care, and the one proving to be the most satisfactory and safe should be used. Bear in mind that the patient will inevitably use his own technique in the end.

NEGOTIATING STEPS AND STAIRS

Handrails or some other firmly fixed supports are needed if the patient is to attempt this activity with his limbs on. Experience has shown that the safest method is for him to stand facing the step or stairs, holding a rail in each hand. By pressing up on to his hands the limbs can be lifted on to the first step. This method is then repeated for each step. It must be remembered that the higher the step, the more difficult it becomes. Coming down is easier. Facing the top step and holding a rail firmly in each hand, the limbs can again be lifted and lowered on to the lower step. The hands must not be placed too far forward, otherwise the body will swing forward and miss the step. It will be clearly obvious that strong upper limbs are essential if this activity is to be safe and practical.

Amputees who fall into this category would normally be advised to consider arranging their home conditions to suit their convenience, even to the extent of having their bedroom, toilet etc. on the ground floor. This, however, should not prevent the patient from being able to negotiate steps and stairs. He should be taught to do this without his limbs, by using one or two hand blocks.

Should any patient in this category be so unfortunate as to fall, he might be expected to be too shocked to make any attempt at getting up off the floor without some assistance. It is indeed advisable that two other people help lift him on to his limbs again, provided that those concerned can confirm that he is in fact fit to continue wearing his limbs, having sustained no personal injury, and that the limbs have not been damaged and are safe to use. The simplest and safest suggestion is that the limbs should be taken off and the patient rested.

# Index

# Index